# The Neuro-Affirming Midwife

## Practical Care for Autistic & ADHD Parents from Pregnancy to Postnatal

I0039723

**Avery Shayla Lawrence**

**Disclaimers**

This book provides **educational information** for midwifery and maternity professionals. It is **not** medical advice, legal advice, or a clinical protocol. Readers must follow local laws, professional codes, employer policies, and current clinical guidelines. Clinical decisions remain the responsibility of the clinician and care team.

Care suggestions are intended to support, not replace, professional judgement. Always assess individual needs and consult senior clinicians as required. Medication, anaesthesia, and surgical decisions rest with appropriately trained and authorised practitioners.

Any case examples use composite scenarios. Names, ages, timelines, and identifying details have been changed to protect privacy. Any resemblance to actual persons, living or dead, is coincidental.

References to organisations, agencies, brands, tools, or guidelines (for example, NHS, NICE, RCOG, or others) are for **identification only**. This publication is **not affiliated with, sponsored by, or endorsed by** any third party. All trademarks remain the property of their respective owners.

Templates, scripts, and checklists are **examples**. Adapt for local policy, documentation standards, and the individual's consent preferences before use.

# The Invisible Intersection

You probably became a midwife because you care. Deeply. You wanted to support people during one of the most intense, vulnerable, and incredible times of their lives. You're good at reading the room, offering a steady hand, and navigating the unpredictable nature of birth. You know how to connect.

But what happens when the person you are trying to connect with experiences the world in a fundamentally different way? What if the standard ways you show care—making eye contact, using a soft voice, offering a reassuring touch—actually cause distress?

Think about a recent shift. Maybe you had a client who seemed distant, almost cold. She avoided eye contact, flinched when the blood pressure cuff inflated, and gave one-word answers to your questions. You might have thought she was anxious, or perhaps just difficult. You tried harder, talked more, maybe even moved closer. And she shut down completely.

Or perhaps you cared for someone who couldn't sit still during a prenatal appointment. She interrupted you constantly, asked a million questions about things that seemed irrelevant, and probably forgot half of what you told her by the time she reached the parking lot. You might have felt frustrated, rushed, and worried she wasn't taking things seriously.

Here's the deal. These aren't examples of difficult patients. These are often examples of unsupported neurodivergence.

We are standing at an invisible intersection. It's where the established practices of midwifery meet the rapidly growing understanding of the human brain. For too long, we've designed maternity services for the "neurotypical" majority—those whose brains process information and sensory input in the way society expects. And in doing so, we have unintentionally marginalized a significant portion of the people giving birth. This book is about making that intersection visible. It's about changing our practices so that every parent, regardless of their neurology, receives safe, respectful, and affirming care.

## The numbers demand our attention

Let's look at the reality on the ground. When we talk about neurodiversity, we're talking about a substantial part of the population. The term neurodiversity includes conditions like Autism, ADHD (Attention Deficit Hyperactivity Disorder), dyslexia, dyspraxia, and others. These aren't rare occurrences.

Current estimates suggest that up to 15% of the population is neurodiverse (British Journal of Midwifery, 2024). Think about that for a second. Fifteen percent.

Let's break down what that means for your daily work. If you work in a busy unit seeing 20 clients in a day, statistically, three of those clients are likely neurodivergent. If your service delivers 5,000 babies a year, around 750 of those parents might be Autistic, have ADHD, or another neurodivergent condition.

These numbers are huge. And honestly? They are probably underestimated.

For decades, Autism and ADHD were seen primarily as conditions affecting young boys. The diagnostic criteria were based on how males present. This means countless women and assigned female at birth (AFAB) individuals have slipped through the net. They learned to "mask"—to hide their traits, suppress their natural responses, and try to fit into a neurotypical world. It's exhausting. Truly exhausting. And it often leads to severe anxiety, depression, and burnout.

Here's where it gets really interesting for us as midwives. Many people don't realize they are neurodivergent until they become pregnant (Maternal Mental Health Alliance, 2025).

Why? Well, pregnancy changes everything. The hormonal shifts, the sensory intensity of the physical changes, the overwhelming demands of planning and appointments—it can crack the mask wide open. The coping mechanisms that worked before suddenly fail. The structure they relied on disappears.

So, when you meet a client for the first time, you are often meeting someone who is not only navigating the massive transition to parenthood but also grappling with a new understanding of their own brain. Or, they might not have a diagnosis at all. They just know they feel overwhelmed, misunderstood, and terrified of the birth experience.

The implication for midwifery is clear. This is not a niche issue. It's a mainstream issue. We can no longer treat neurodiversity-affirming care as an optional extra or something only specialists do. It must be woven into the fabric of everything we do.

**We have a critical need and a call to action**

The profession is waking up to this reality. The leadership knows we need to do better. In 2024, the Royal College of Midwives (RCM) issued new guidance highlighting the critical need for specialized support for neurodivergent parents (Royal College of Midwives, 2024). And this isn't just happening in one country; the conversation is global.

This guidance isn't just a quiet suggestion. It's a mandate for change. It recognizes that the current system is failing these parents and that midwives are on the front line of making the necessary adjustments.

The professional guidance emphasizes several key areas:

1. **Recognition:** We need to get better at recognizing the signs of neurodivergence, even without a formal diagnosis. It's about observing needs, not diagnosing conditions.

2. **Communication:** We must adapt how we communicate information, moving away from abstract language and ensuring clarity and processing time.

3. **Environment:** The sensory environment of maternity units is often hostile to neurodivergent people. The lights, the sounds, the textures—we need to address this urgently.

4. **Choice and Control:** Neurodivergent individuals need genuine choice and control over their care, which requires predictable pathways and personalized support.

Research echoes this urgency. Studies have shown a "critical need for neurodiversity-affirming practices" in maternity care (Hampton et al., 2022). This research highlights that when we don't adapt our care, we risk causing significant harm.

Why now? The convergence of increased awareness, better diagnostic tools (though still imperfect), and a powerful self-advocacy movement driven by neurodivergent adults means we can no longer ignore the issue. People are speaking up about their experiences. They are demanding better.

And frankly, it's about basic human rights and legal obligations. Laws like the Americans with Disabilities Act (ADA) in the US, or the Equality Act in the UK, require public services to make "reasonable accommodations" or adjustments for disabled people. Autism and ADHD are recognized disabilities. So, providing adapted care isn't just good practice; it's often a legal requirement.

Think of it like this: If a patient needed a wheelchair, you wouldn't ask them to try harder to walk up the stairs. You would find a ramp. Neurodiversity-affirming care is the ramp. It's about providing the necessary adjustments so everyone can access the care they deserve.

But let's put the legal stuff aside for a moment. It's about our professional ethics. As midwives, we are committed to providing individualized, person-centered care. How can we claim to do that if we are ignoring the fundamental neurology of 15% of our clients? We can't.

The mandate is clear. We have the guidance. We have the evidence. Now we need the practical skills.

## The cost of getting it wrong is high

Let's talk about what happens when we don't adapt our care. The consequences of unsupported care are severe and long-lasting. This isn't just about making people feel comfortable, although that is very important. It's about safety, engagement, and equity.

**Trauma is the biggest risk.** The birth experience is inherently intense. For someone with sensory processing differences, the standard birth environment can be agonizing. The bright fluorescent lights, the constant beeping of machines, the unfamiliar smells, the intrusion of strangers, the feeling of the fetal monitor straps—it can be overwhelming.

When a neurodivergent person is overwhelmed, they can enter a state of sensory overload. This isn't just stress. It can lead to a meltdown or a shutdown.

A meltdown might look like extreme distress, crying, yelling, or even aggression. It's an outward expression of "I can't cope." It is not a tantrum. It is an involuntary response to distress.

A shutdown is often quieter but just as serious. The person might become non-verbal, retreat inward, and be unable to process information or make decisions. They might look compliant, but they are actually frozen in fear.

When this happens during labor, the consequences are profound. The physiological process of labor can stall. The need for interventions increases. And the experience is coded in the brain as trauma.

Consider Sarah's story. Sarah is Autistic, though she didn't know it when she had her first baby. She arrived at the hospital in labor and was immediately put into a bright triage room. The midwife, rushed and distracted (we've all been there), asked her questions rapidly while attaching monitors. Sarah felt the walls closing in. She tried to explain she needed the lights dimmed, but the midwife said it was policy to keep them on for observation.

When the midwife performed a vaginal examination without explicit warning, Sarah experienced it as an assault. She shut down. She couldn't communicate her pain levels or her needs. Her labor stalled, leading to a cascade of interventions and eventually an emergency Cesarean section. Sarah developed severe postnatal depression and PTSD. She felt she had failed at birth. But the truth is, the system failed Sarah.

This kind of trauma has lasting effects. It impacts bonding with the baby. It increases the risk of perinatal mental health problems. And it makes people afraid to seek healthcare in the future.

**Poor engagement is another consequence.** Prenatal care relies on regular attendance and open communication. If appointments are stressful, confusing, or overwhelming, neurodivergent parents may disengage.

Think about someone with ADHD. They may struggle with executive functioning—the mental processes that help us plan, organize, and manage time. Remembering appointments, filling out forms, and following complex instructions can be incredibly difficult. If they miss an appointment and are met with judgment or impatience, they are less likely to come back. We might label them "non-compliant," but often, they are just unsupported.

This disengagement means missed opportunities for screening, education, and support. It can lead to adverse outcomes for both the parent and the baby.

**Health inequalities are the result.** Neurodivergent people already face significant health inequalities across the board. They often have co-occurring conditions, such as anxiety, depression, and chronic physical health issues (like Ehlers-Danlos Syndrome). In maternity care, these inequalities are magnified.

Research suggests that Autistic parents are more likely to experience induced labor, instrumental birth, and Cesarean sections (Sundelin et al. 2018). They are also less satisfied with their care and report higher levels of birth trauma.

This isn't because their bodies are less capable of giving birth. It's because the system is not set up to support them. We are creating a situation where one group of people, simply because of their neurology, receives substandard care and experiences worse outcomes. That is the definition of inequality. And it is unacceptable.

**This book is a toolkit for change**

When I first started looking into this topic, I felt overwhelmed. I realized how many mistakes I had made, how many times I had misunderstood a client's behavior, and how many opportunities I had missed to provide truly affirming care. It's tough to realize you might have unintentionally caused harm. (It's a realization we all have to face.)

I looked for resources. I searched for books that would give me practical guidance on how to support Autistic and ADHD parents during pregnancy, labor, and the postnatal period. You know what I found? Almost nothing.

There are excellent books on neurodiversity. There are excellent books on midwifery. But there was very little that connected the two in a practical way. There was no toolkit for the busy midwife on the floor at 3 AM who needs to know how to adapt their care right now.

That's why this book exists.

The purpose of this book is to provide you with that practical toolkit. It's designed to be clear, accessible, and immediately applicable to your practice, whether you work in the community, on the prenatal ward, in a birth center, or on the labor ward.

This book will help you:

- **Understand** the lived experience of Autism and ADHD during the perinatal period.

- **Recognize** the signs of neurodivergence, even when masked.

- **Adapt** your communication strategies to meet the needs of neurodiverse clients.

- **Modify** the sensory environment to create a safe and supportive space.

- **Support** neurodivergent parents through the challenges of labor, birth, and the postnatal period.

- **Advocate** for systemic change within your maternity service.

This isn't about becoming a neurodiversity expert overnight. It's about making small, manageable changes that have a massive impact. It's about shifting your perspective from a deficit model (what's wrong with this person?) to a difference model (how does this person experience the world, and how can I support them?).

We will use real-life case examples (like Sarah's) to illustrate the concepts and strategies. We will provide checklists, templates, and scripts you can use in your daily practice. And we will do it in a way that is respectful, affirming, and empowering for both you and the families you care for.

Are you ready? Good. Let's get started on making midwifery truly inclusive.

**The words we use matter**

Before we go any further, we need to talk about language. This part is crucial. The words we use to describe neurodiversity and neurodivergent people matter. A lot. Language shapes our attitudes, our beliefs, and ultimately, our actions.

Historically, the "medical model" has used language that is deficit-focused. It talks about disorders, impairments, and deficits. It implies that neurodivergent people are broken and need to be fixed.

The neurodiversity movement, which is led by neurodivergent people themselves, rejects this model. It embraces the "neurodiversity paradigm," which views neurodiversity as a natural form of human variation. There is no one "right" type of brain. This aligns closely with the "social model" of disability, which argues that people are disabled by barriers in society (like inaccessible environments or rigid procedures), not by their bodies or brains.

As midwives, it is crucial that we adopt respectful, identity-affirming language. This shows our clients that we see them, we respect them, and we are committed to providing supportive care.

Here is a guide to some key terms and concepts.

**Neurodiversity vs Neurodivergence vs Neurotypical**

This can be confusing, so let's break it down simply. (It took me a while to get this straight too.)

- **Neurodiversity** is a broad term that refers to the diversity of human brains within a group of people. It's like biodiversity. A group can be neurodiverse (containing people with different types of brains), but an individual cannot be neurodiverse.

- **Neurodivergent (ND)** is the term used to describe an individual whose brain functions differently from what society considers standard or typical. This includes Autism, ADHD, dyslexia, dyspraxia, Tourette syndrome, and others.

- **Neurotypical (NT)** is the term used to describe an individual whose brain functions in the way society expects.

So, you might say: "We are committed to supporting **neurodivergent** clients as part of the natural **neurodiversity** of our population."

**Identity-First Language (IFL) vs Person-First Language (PFL)**

This is a big one, especially when talking about Autism.

- **Person-First Language (PFL)** puts the person before the condition. For example, "person with autism" or "person who has ADHD."

- **Identity-First Language (IFL)** puts the identity first. For example, "Autistic person" or "ADHDer."

For many years, healthcare professionals were taught to always use PFL. The idea was to emphasize the personhood of the individual. And that's well-intentioned.

However, the majority of the Autistic community prefers IFL (Kenny et al., 2016). Why? Because Autism is not something they *have*. It's something they *are*. It is an inseparable part of their identity and how they experience the world.

Saying "person with autism" implies that autism is a negative add-on that can or should be removed. Saying "Autistic person" acknowledges that autism is a core part of their identity.

As one Autistic advocate put it, you wouldn't say "person with femaleness" or "person with gayness." You would say "woman" or "gay person." It's an identity.

When it comes to ADHD, preferences are more mixed. Some prefer "person with ADHD," while others prefer "ADHDer" or simply saying "I have ADHD."

So, what should you do?

1. **Default to IFL for Autism.** Use "Autistic person" unless the individual tells you otherwise.

2. **Be flexible with ADHD.** You can use "person with ADHD" or "ADHD parent."

3. **Listen and respect.** The most important thing is to listen to how the person refers to themselves and respect their preference. If you aren't sure, just ask! "How would you like me to refer to your neurodivergence?"

### Avoiding Ableist Language

Ableist language is language that discriminates against disabled people. It often frames disability as negative, tragic, or something to be overcome. We need to be mindful of this in our practice and documentation.

Here are some examples of ableist language to avoid and what to use instead:

- **Instead of:** "Suffering from autism" or "A victim of ADHD."

- **Use:** "Is Autistic" or "Has ADHD."

- **Instead of:** "High-functioning" or "Low-functioning." (These terms are deeply problematic. They ignore the spectrum of strengths and challenges a person may have, and they often invalidate the struggles of those deemed "high-functioning.")

- **Use:** Describe the person's specific support needs. For example, "Requires support with communication" or "Needs a low-sensory environment."

- **Instead of:** "Special needs."

- **Use:** "Specific needs," "Support needs," or "Disability." The term "special needs" can be seen as patronizing.

**Understanding Key Concepts**

Let's quickly define a few other terms we will use throughout this book:

- **Stimming:** Short for self-stimulatory behavior. It refers to repetitive movements, sounds, or actions (like hand-flapping, rocking, humming, repeating phrases, or using a fidget toy) that neurodivergent people use to regulate their emotions, cope with sensory input, or express themselves. Stimming is not a problem to be stopped. It is a necessary and healthy coping mechanism. In the context of birth, stimming is incredibly important for managing pain and anxiety. We need to recognize and support it.

- **Meltdowns and Shutdowns:** We talked about these earlier, but let's be clear. A meltdown or shutdown is an involuntary response to overwhelm (sensory, emotional, or informational). It is not a tantrum. It is not manipulative behavior. It is a sign that the person is in extreme distress and needs support.

- **Masking:** Masking, also known as camouflaging, is the conscious or unconscious suppression of one's natural traits and behaviors to fit into neurotypical expectations. It is common in Autistic people and those with ADHD, especially those diagnosed later in life. Masking is exhausting and has a significant impact on mental health.

By adopting respectful and accurate language, we create a foundation of trust and safety. It signals to our neurodivergent clients that we are allies. It shows that we are willing to learn and adapt our practice to meet their needs. It might feel tricky at first, and that's okay. The effort matters more than perfection.

This journey starts with understanding the landscape we are in—the prevalence, the need, the risks, and the language. In the next part of the book, we will begin building the foundations of neuro-affirming midwifery, starting with a deeper look at what neurodivergence actually means in the perinatal context.

---

**What You've Learned**

- Neurodiversity is common. Up to 15% of the population is neurodiverse, meaning a significant portion of the clients you see are likely Autistic, have ADHD, or another neurodivergent condition.

- Many people are not diagnosed until pregnancy, often because they have been masking their traits. Pregnancy makes this specialized support essential.

- Professional organizations recognize the critical need for neurodiversity-affirming practices. This is a mandate for change in midwifery.

- The consequences of unsupported care are severe, including birth trauma (often stemming from sensory overload and communication barriers), poor engagement with services, adverse outcomes, and increased health inequalities.

- This book provides a practical toolkit for midwives to adapt their communication, environment, and care strategies to support neurodivergent parents.

- Language matters. Using respectful, identity-affirming language (such as "Autistic person" instead of "person with autism") is crucial for building trust and providing affirming care.

- Understanding key concepts like the neurodiversity paradigm, stimming, meltdowns, shutdowns, and masking is foundational to this work.

# Chapter 1: Neurodivergence in the Perinatal Context

When we meet a new person, our brains immediately start putting together a profile. We listen to how they talk, we watch their body language, we notice if they make eye contact. We do this to understand them. It's what we've been trained to do. But what if the way you read someone is based on a set of rules that don't apply to them? What if the person in front of you is operating with a completely different operating system?

This is the reality of caring for neurodivergent individuals. Their brains are wired differently. They aren't broken, they just work another way. Before we can provide true, affirming care, we have to understand the basics of this different wiring. We have to learn to read the signs and re-evaluate our assumptions. This chapter is your foundation. It's where we get into the nuts and bolts of what Autism and ADHD can look like in adults, especially in the context of pregnancy and birth.

## Defining the spectrum: Autism and ADHD

We'll focus on Autism and ADHD because they are the most common forms of neurodivergence we will encounter in maternity care. It's helpful to think of both as a spectrum, not a checklist. You can't be "a little bit Autistic." You are or you aren't. But the way it shows up can be a million different shades.

**Autism** is a lifelong developmental condition that affects how a person communicates, interacts with others, and experiences the world.[1]

Key traits often include:

- **Differences in social communication and interaction:** This doesn't mean a person is shy or antisocial. It means they may struggle with things like unspoken social rules, reading facial expressions, or making small talk. They might prefer direct, factual conversation over social pleasantries.

- **Restricted, repetitive behaviors and interests:** This can look like needing a specific routine, having intense and focused interests (sometimes called "special interests"), or engaging in repetitive movements (stimming) to self-soothe.

- **Sensory processing differences:** A person might be either hyper-sensitive (overly sensitive) or hypo-sensitive (under-sensitive) to sensory input like sound, light, touch, or smell.[2]

**ADHD** (Attention Deficit Hyperactivity Disorder) is a neurodevelopmental condition that affects a person's ability to regulate attention, manage their emotions, and control their impulses.[3] It's not about a lack of attention; it's about a lack of control over where that attention goes.

Key traits often include:

- **Inattention:** This can look like being easily distracted, struggling to follow multi-step instructions, forgetting appointments, and losing things. It's often misunderstood as laziness or disorganization.

- **Hyperactivity and Impulsivity:** For many, especially adults, this isn't physical restlessness. It's an internal restlessness—a buzzing feeling in the brain. It can show up as being talkative, interrupting others, and making impulsive decisions.

It's important to know that many people have both. The conditions can and do overlap. ADHD traits can mask Autistic ones, and vice versa. It's a complex puzzle, but the goal isn't for you to figure out the diagnosis. The goal is to recognize a pattern of needs and provide the right support.

**The Female Phenotype and Masking: Why many go undiagnosed**

Here's a major reason why you're encountering so many undiagnosed people. Historically, the diagnostic criteria for Autism and ADHD were based almost entirely on how they present in young boys (Lai et al., 2015). The traits of hyperactive little boys who couldn't sit still in a classroom or who were socially withdrawn were the ones we learned to look for.

Turns out, girls and AFAB individuals (assigned female at birth) often present very differently.[4] This is sometimes called the **female phenotype**.

For example, Autistic women may be less likely to have obvious, outward stims. Instead of hand-flapping, they might have a subtle stim like playing with a ring on their finger or biting the inside of their cheek.

Socially, instead of being withdrawn, they might be highly motivated to fit in. They study their peers, analyze social situations, and mimic what others do. This is called **masking**, and it's exhausting.[5] (Imagine trying to act like a person from a different country every single minute of your life.) They learn what to say, what expressions to make, and what not to do to avoid standing out. And they get very, very good at it.

Masking is a survival strategy. The person with ADHD or Autism learns that their natural way of being is unacceptable, so they hide it.[6] But hiding a core part of who you are has a steep price. Over time, it leads to severe anxiety, depression, burnout, and a deep sense of not belonging.

Pregnancy is a time when the mask often slips. The hormonal changes, the physical discomfort, and the sheer unpredictability of it all can be too much to maintain the facade. The person who seemed perfectly "normal" during their first trimester might show up for a later appointment visibly struggling. And you might be the first person to witness it.

Think of Sarah again, the client from the introduction. She was an accomplished professional. She had friends and a partner. On the outside, she was a success story. She was good at masking. But pregnancy shattered her carefully constructed routine. She couldn't control her body or her schedule, and the constant flux was terrifying. Her mask cracked, and she was left with nothing to protect her from the overwhelming sensory experience of her own body and the world.

So, when a client is struggling, don't just see anxiety. Ask yourself, "Could this be masking that has reached its limit?"

### Executive Functioning: The brain's control tower

To really understand ADHD and Autism, you have to understand **executive functioning**. This is the brain's set of mental skills that help us get things done. Think of it as the control tower of your brain. It helps you:

- **Plan and organize:** Breaking a big task (like preparing for a baby) into small steps.

- **Initiate tasks:** Actually starting a task.

- **Prioritize:** Deciding what's most important.

- **Manage time:** Knowing how long a task will take and sticking to a schedule.

- **Work with memory:** Holding information in your mind while you work on it.

- **Regulate emotions:** Controlling your reactions to things.

For people with ADHD and often with Autism, the control tower isn't working at full power. It's not that they don't want to do something; it's that the brain's "on" switch is broken. They can know exactly what they need to do, but they can't make themselves do it. This is sometimes called **ADHD paralysis**.

How does this play out in the perinatal period?

- **Antenatal appointments:** A parent with ADHD might struggle to remember appointment times, bring the correct paperwork, or recall instructions you gave them. This isn't disrespect; it's a breakdown in their planning and working memory.

- **Birth planning:** Creating a birth plan requires a lot of executive function—researching options, making decisions, and writing it down. This can feel impossible.

- **Postpartum:** The demands of a newborn are a massive executive functioning challenge. The constant need for feeding, diaper changes, and lack of sleep can completely break a person who already struggles with these skills. This is a primary reason why postnatal depression rates are higher in neurodivergent parents (Farr et al., 2023).

When you see a client who seems disorganized or forgetful, try not to get frustrated. Instead, shift your approach. Use simple checklists. Set a reminder for them. Send information in a text message or a short email. Be their external executive function. It's a simple change that makes a massive difference.

### Sensory Processing Differences: The world is too much

Imagine you are in a room with a buzzing fluorescent light. You hear every single beep of the machines down the hall. The texture of the paper on the bed is scratchy against your skin. The smell of the hospital hand sanitizer is overpowering. Now, multiply all of that by ten. That's a day in the life of someone with **sensory hypersensitivity**.

Or, what if you barely feel pain? You get a cut on your hand and don't notice it. You feel pressure, but you don't feel touch. This is **hyposensitivity**.

For neurodivergent individuals, the way their brain processes sensory information can be very different from the norm.[7] It's not just a matter of preference. It's a matter of neurological wiring.

- **Hypersensitivity:** This is when the nervous system is flooded with sensory input. Everything is too loud, too bright, too smelly, too scratchy. This is a common reason for meltdowns. During labor, the sensory input is intense: the pain of contractions, the bright lights of the labor ward, the sounds of others, the touch of a midwife.[8] For someone who is hypersensitive, this can be unbearable and lead to a physical shutdown of the body.

- **Hyposensitivity:** This is when the nervous system needs more input to register something. A person with hyposensitivity might seek out strong sensory experiences. During labor, this could mean they don't seem to feel or respond to contractions in a typical way. They may need strong, firm pressure to feel touch or they may not recognize when they need to push.

It's easy to misunderstand this. A client who flinches when you touch them isn't rejecting you. They are reacting to an unexpected and overwhelming sensation. A client who seems "unbothered" by labor pain isn't just tough; their brain might be processing the pain signals differently.

Understanding this is your key to providing affirming care. The answer isn't to force them to tolerate the standard environment. The answer is to adapt the environment for them. We will talk all about that in a later chapter. But first, you have to know what you're looking for.

### The Neurodiversity Paradigm: Shifting from a deficit to a difference

This is the most important idea in this chapter. It's the framework that should guide all of your actions. For years, medicine has operated from a **deficit model**. It sees neurodivergence as a problem to be fixed, a disease to be cured, or a deficit to be overcome. It focuses on what is "wrong" with the person and how to make them "normal."

The **neurodiversity paradigm** rejects this idea completely. It sees neurodiversity as a natural, healthy, and valuable form of human variation (Walker, 2021). Just like we have different eye colors, we have different brain wirings. Neither is better or worse; they are simply different.

This shift in perspective is everything. It changes your questions.

- Instead of asking, "Why is this person being so difficult?" you ask, **"What needs are not being met here?"**

- Instead of asking, "How can I fix this person's communication issues?" you ask, **"How can I change my communication style to connect with this person?"**

- Instead of asking, "Why can't she handle this?" you ask, **"What adjustments can I make so she can thrive?"**

This isn't just about being nice. This is about providing better, safer care. When we operate from a difference model, we stop trying to force square pegs into round holes. We start building square holes. This is the truth. It's the only way we can ensure everyone gets the care they deserve.

This shift is crucial for you, too. When you stop seeing your client's behaviors as defiance or difficulty and start seeing them as a response to an environment that isn't built for them, your frustration disappears. It is replaced with empathy and a sense of purpose. And that, my friend, is what midwifery is all about.

# Chapter 2: The Neurodivergent Experience of Pregnancy and Birth

Now that we've got the basics down, let's get into the heart of it. What is it actually like to be Autistic or have ADHD while your body is going through the immense changes of pregnancy and birth? What we'll see here is that neurodivergence doesn't just add a layer of complexity; it completely changes the game.

**The impact of hormonal shifts on Autistic and ADHD traits**

You know how pregnancy hormones can cause mood swings and brain fog in anyone? Well, for someone who is already navigating a nervous system that struggles with regulation, hormonal shifts are like throwing gasoline on a fire.

For someone with ADHD, the lack of dopamine and norepinephrine can be a huge issue. These are the chemicals that help with focus, motivation, and emotional regulation. During pregnancy, hormonal changes can disrupt the delicate balance of these neurotransmitters. This can lead to an increase in ADHD symptoms: the brain fog gets thicker, the forgetfulness gets worse, and the emotional dysregulation can become extreme. Rejection Sensitive Dysphoria (RSD), which we'll discuss in a moment, can spike. The pregnant person might feel completely out of control of their own thoughts and emotions.

For Autistic people, hormonal changes can intensify sensory sensitivities and change their capacity for masking. For some, the new smells and textures of their own body become overwhelming. The nausea of morning sickness can feel like a sensory assault. Their carefully constructed routines can be completely disrupted, leading to increased anxiety and distress. The energy they once had to mask might be gone, leading to more frequent meltdowns or shutdowns. A lot of the time, the pregnant person isn't really sure why they are suddenly struggling so much, because they don't yet have the language to connect it to their neurodivergence.

**Interoception Challenges: What is my body even doing?**

This next part is fascinating, and it's a huge reason why birth can be so difficult for some neurodivergent people.

**Interoception** is the sense of what's happening inside your body. It's how your brain understands signals like hunger, thirst, pain, needing to go to the bathroom, or feeling too hot or too cold. It's the quiet conversation between your brain and your body.

For many Autistic people, that conversation is either muffled or completely garbled (Hampton et al.,2023). They might be **hyposensitive** to interoceptive signals, meaning they don't feel them strongly. A person might not feel hunger until they are starving, or thirst until they are dehydrated.

Or, they might be **hypersensitive**, meaning the signals are so loud and overwhelming that they are impossible to distinguish. A stomachache could feel like a full-blown emergency.

How does this affect pregnancy and birth? This is huge.

- **Early labor:** A person with interoception challenges might not recognize early labor signs. They may not feel the contractions until they are intense and close together. They might not realize they are in active labor until they are far progressed. This can lead to arriving at the hospital later than planned, which is a common source of anxiety and frustration for both the person and the care team.

- **Pain management:** A person who is hyposensitive to pain might have a high pain tolerance, so they might not ask for pain relief when they need it. A person who is hypersensitive to pain might experience contractions as completely unbearable. In both cases, the standard pain scale (the one we use all the time) can be meaningless.

- **Postpartum:** The signs of postpartum hemorrhage, like lightheadedness or a racing heart, might not be felt. Or, a person might not recognize the need to use the bathroom until it's an emergency. This is a safety issue.

So, instead of relying on the standard "how are you feeling on a scale of 1 to 10?" question, you need to rely on objective observations and creative communication. Instead of asking "Are you hungry?" you might say, "It's been four hours since you last ate. Let's get a snack."

## Communication Differences: Literal vs. inferred

Midwifery is built on communication. We give instructions, we provide information, we offer reassurance. But what if the person you're talking to understands words in a completely literal way?

For many Autistic people, literal interpretation is the default. They hear exactly what you say, not what you mean.

Let's say you tell a client, "Don't worry, you'll be fine." To a neurotypical person, this is a kind reassurance. To a literal thinker, it's a confusing command. They might think, "Why are you telling me not to worry? Is there something I should be worrying about? And what does 'fine' even mean?"

This is part of something called the **Double Empathy Problem** (Milton, 2012).[9] It's the idea that communication difficulties between Autistic and non-Autistic people are not caused by a deficit in the Autistic person, but by a mismatch in communication styles.[10] It's a two-way street. We struggle to understand them, just as they struggle to understand us.

Another key piece of this is **processing time**. A neurotypical person can often hear a question and answer it immediately. Many neurodivergent people need more time to process information. They might need a few seconds, or even a few minutes, to think about what you said, organize their thoughts, and formulate a response. If you don't give them this time and jump in with more questions, you can cause a lot of anxiety and confusion.

Look, this is not just an inconvenience. It can lead to serious errors. A client who says "yes" to your question because they are overwhelmed and want to move on might not have understood what they just consented to.

**Emotional Regulation: The rollercoaster ride**

Emotional regulation is the ability to manage and respond to an emotional experience. It's a huge challenge for many neurodivergent people.

We talked about meltdowns and shutdowns in the introduction. A meltdown is an external expression of overwhelm. It can look like yelling, crying, or lashing out. A shutdown is an internal collapse. The person becomes quiet, withdrawn, and may seem "blank."

**Rejection Sensitive Dysphoria (RSD)** is a common and very painful experience for people with ADHD (Doodson, 2022). It's an extreme emotional sensitivity and pain triggered by the perception of being rejected, criticized, or teased.[11] The pain is as intense as a physical injury.

How does this affect care?

- **Meltdowns/Shutdowns:** During labor, pain and sensory overload can trigger a meltdown. You might have a client who is suddenly screaming or completely non-responsive. The standard medical response is to get the person to calm down, but what they really need is to have the overwhelming stimuli removed.

- **RSD:** A midwife's well-intentioned but poorly phrased comment can trigger an intense RSD response. Say you say, "You really should have brought your birth plan with you." To you, it's a gentle prompt. To a person with RSD, it sounds like, "You are a failure. You messed up. I am disappointed in you."

This can cause a sudden, intense flood of shame and pain, making them withdraw or lash out.

Understanding these emotional experiences means we can respond with compassion and not judgment. We can learn to rephrase our language to avoid perceived criticism and to offer a safe, non-judgmental space.

## Co-occurring conditions and intersectionality

The neurodivergent experience is rarely one-dimensional. Many conditions often appear together, which is called **co-occurring conditions** or **comorbidity**.[12] This is incredibly common and important for you to be aware of.

For example, many Autistic people have Ehlers-Danlos Syndrome (EDS), a connective tissue disorder that affects joints and skin (Casanova et al., 2020).[13] This can mean increased joint pain, stretchy skin, and a high risk of injury during birth. A person with both Autism and EDS might have challenges with interoception and also have physical pain that is not immediately visible.

Mental health conditions are also highly co-occurring.[14] Anxiety, depression, and eating disorders are much more prevalent in neurodivergent people. And we know that the perinatal period is already a time of increased risk for these conditions.[15]

We also have to think about **intersectionality**. This is the idea that a person's identity is made up of multiple, overlapping social categories (like race, gender, class, and neurodivergence). This creates unique experiences of discrimination and privilege.

For example, a Black Autistic person might face not only ableism but also systemic racism within the healthcare system. The combination of these biases can lead to a severely degraded standard of care. We have to be aware of these layers and work to provide care that is not only neuro-affirming but also culturally humble and anti-racist.

The goal here isn't to diagnose a person with all of their co-occurring conditions. The goal is to understand that what you see on the surface—the anxiety, the pain, the physical symptoms—might be linked to something deeper. And that by addressing the core neurodivergent needs, you can often provide a solution for many of the co-occurring challenges.

This chapter might feel heavy. But it's necessary. It's the lens through which you must view everything else in this book. Once you can see the world through the neurodivergent experience, your path forward becomes clear. It's a path of empathy, adaptation, and affirmation.

# Chapter 3: Principles of Trauma-Informed and Affirming Practice

So, we've established that neurodivergent people are common in our care and that their experiences of pregnancy and birth are fundamentally different.[16] Now we have to talk about how we respond to that. We can't just stand there and watch; we have to act. This chapter is about the "how." It's about building a framework for care that is safe, ethical, and truly person-centered.

**The link between standard care and trauma**

We have to be honest with ourselves. Standard maternity care is often not trauma-informed for neurodivergent individuals. In fact, it can be actively traumatic. Our systems are built for efficiency, not for personalized sensory and communication needs.

Think about a typical labor ward. The bright lights, the constant chatter, the beeping of machines, the smell of disinfectant, the repeated questions from different providers—it's a sensory nightmare. The neurodivergent brain, which struggles to filter out this noise, becomes overwhelmed.

Then there are the procedures. An unscheduled vaginal examination with no clear warning or explanation can feel like a violation of personal space. The need for constant monitoring can be physically and emotionally restrictive. The lack of control over one's own body and the process can be terrifying. A person with executive functioning challenges might be told to "just relax" when their brain is actively fighting against them.

This isn't about bad intentions. This is about a system that is unintentionally harmful. Midwives are not trying to be traumatic. But our systems and our standard practices can be. And for a neurodivergent person, this can lead to what's called **iatrogenic trauma**—trauma caused by the healthcare system itself. The birth experience, instead of being a rite of passage, becomes an assault on their senses and their autonomy.

We have a duty to stop this.

**Core principles of Trauma-Informed Care**

Trauma-informed care is a model that understands how trauma affects people and aims to avoid re-traumatization. It's a perfect fit for neuro-affirming midwifery because the things that prevent trauma for neurodivergent people are often the very same things we should be doing for everyone.

The core principles of trauma-informed care are (SAMHSA, 2014):

1. **Safety:** Both physical and emotional safety are paramount. For neurodivergent people, this means creating a predictable and low-sensory environment.[17] It means being transparent about what you are doing and why.

2. **Trustworthiness and Transparency:** Be clear and honest about what to expect. Don't make promises you can't keep. Explain every procedure before you do it, and be honest about the risks and benefits.

3. **Choice:** Give the person a real choice whenever possible. "You have the option to have this fetal monitor on continuously or intermittently. Which would you prefer?" Giving choices helps restore a sense of control that is often lost in a hospital setting.

4. **Collaboration:** Work *with* the person, not *on* them. Ask, "What do you think would be most helpful right now?" Listen to their ideas, even if they seem unconventional. They are the expert on their own body.

5. **Empowerment:** Give the person the tools and knowledge to make their own decisions. Celebrate their strengths. Acknowledge the challenges they are facing. Your role is to support them, not to take over.

These principles are not just for people who have a history of trauma. They are good practice for everyone. They help create a space where your client can feel safe, respected, and heard. And when a neurodivergent person feels safe, their nervous system calms down, and they can engage with their care.

### Legal and ethical obligations: "Reasonable Adjustments"

As a healthcare professional, you have a legal and ethical obligation to provide accessible care. In many countries, like the UK under the Equality Act of 2010, this is a legal requirement. The law requires service providers to make **"reasonable adjustments"** to ensure that disabled people are not put at a "substantial disadvantage" (Equality Act, 2010).[18]

Autism and ADHD are considered disabilities under this law. This means you are legally obligated to make reasonable adjustments for a neurodivergent person in your care.

What counts as a "reasonable adjustment"?

- **Environmental adjustments:** Dimming the lights, providing a quiet room, or offering a fan for temperature regulation.[19]

- **Communication adjustments:** Providing written information, giving more time to process questions, and using simple, literal language.

- **Procedural adjustments:** Bundling care to minimize interruptions, or offering a choice about when to have a procedure.

The truth is, most reasonable adjustments don't cost anything. They just require a shift in perspective and a willingness to adapt.

Beyond the legal side, we have an ethical obligation to care for our clients. The Nursing and Midwifery Council (NMC) code of conduct requires us to "preserve the safety of people in [our] care" and to "treat people with dignity and respect" (NMC, 2018). How can we do that if we ignore their neurological differences? We can't. This is about professional integrity. It's about living up to the promise we made when we chose this career.

**The midwife's role as an advocate and ally**

The most powerful role you can play is that of an **advocate and an ally**.

- **Advocacy:** You are the person who can speak up for your client when they can't speak for themselves. This means you might need to say to a colleague, "Please dim the lights. My client has a sensory sensitivity." Or, "She needs a moment to process that information before we move on." You can be the voice that protects your client from a system that might not understand their needs.

- **Allyship:** Being an ally is a conscious choice to support a marginalized group. It means you are not just a neutral observer; you are actively working to make things better. It means you learn the correct language, you listen to neurodivergent people's stories, and you use your position of privilege to fight for change.

This role isn't easy. It can feel like you are pushing against a big, rigid system. But a single midwife making a small adjustment can prevent a lifetime of trauma. A single midwife with a little knowledge can empower a person who has felt powerless their whole life.

Your role is to bridge the gap. You are the one who can take the knowledge we've discussed in these first chapters and put it into action. You can see the person behind the diagnosis, or the person without one. You can listen, learn, and adapt. And that, my friend, is where the real work of midwifery begins. It's an honor to do it.

**Conclusion: A New Way of Seeing**

In these first three chapters, we have laid the groundwork. We've defined neurodivergence, we've explored the unique challenges it presents in the perinatal context, and we've established the ethical and practical principles of affirming care. This isn't about just adding a checklist to your routine. It's about a fundamental shift in how you see and interact with your clients. It's about moving from a place of judgment to a place of understanding. From a place of "what's wrong?" to a place of "what can I do to help?" This is the core of neuro-affirming midwifery, and it is the single most important tool you will acquire in this book.

---

**What You've Learned**

- **Understanding is everything:** Autism and ADHD are spectrums that affect a person's social communication, sensory processing, and executive functioning. The way they present in adults, especially women, is often masked and goes undiagnosed.[20]

- **Pregnancy is a pressure cooker:** Hormonal shifts, interoception challenges, and communication differences can make pregnancy and birth particularly difficult for neurodivergent people.[21] This can lead to increased stress, anxiety, and a higher risk of trauma.

- **Standard care can be harmful:** The rigid, unpredictable, and high-sensory environment of a hospital can be a source of trauma for neurodivergent people.[22] We have a responsibility to adapt our practices to prevent this.

- **Principles for practice:** Adopting a trauma-informed approach, which prioritizes safety, trustworthiness, choice, collaboration, and empowerment, is essential for all clients, especially neurodivergent ones.

- **Your role is to advocate:** As a midwife, you have a legal and ethical duty to make reasonable adjustments and to act as an ally for your clients. This is the most important thing you can do to ensure they receive safe and respectful care.

# Chapter 4: Recognizing Undiagnosed or Undisclosed Neurodivergence

We tend to operate under the assumption that if someone is neurodivergent—autistic, ADHD, dyslexic—they know it, and they will tell us. We expect a neat label on a chart. But in the world of perinatal care, that assumption is often flat wrong. The reality is, a significant portion of the adults walking into our clinics are navigating life with undiagnosed or undisclosed neurodivergence. They have spent years, maybe decades, feeling misunderstood, thinking they are "too sensitive," "disorganized," or just fundamentally different, without knowing why.

This is especially true for those assigned female at birth. The diagnostic criteria we have used for years were heavily biased toward male presentations. Because of this, and because many individuals learn to "mask"—that is, consciously or unconsciously hide their traits to fit in—a huge number slip through the cracks. Some studies suggest that nearly 80% of autistic females might be undiagnosed by the age of 18 (Loomes et al., 2022). Eighty percent. Let that sink in.

So, when we talk about providing neuro-affirming care, we cannot just focus on those with a formal diagnosis. That is the easy part. The real challenge, and the real opportunity for impact, is recognizing that **any** client might be neurodivergent. Our approach must shift from reactive (providing accommodations when asked) to proactive (creating an accessible environment for everyone).

This is not about diagnosing anyone in the clinic. That is not our role. It is about recognizing potential needs and adapting our care immediately. It is about creating safety, whether a diagnosis is present or not.

## Behavioral and communication cues during antenatal appointments

When a pregnant person comes in, they are already vulnerable. Pregnancy is intense—physically, emotionally, and sensorily. For someone who is undiagnosed neurodivergent, the clinical environment can feel downright hostile. The buzzing lights, the beeping machines, the unpredictable waiting times, the social demands—it is a lot to handle.

Their response to this environment, and to you, will often give you clues about their neurology. We need to become keen observers. Put down the checklist for a second and really **look** at the person in front of you.

Understanding the spiky profile

It helps to understand the concept of the "spiky profile." Neurotypical individuals usually have a relatively flat skill profile. They are generally average across the board—communication, organization, sensory processing.

Neurodivergent individuals often have a "spiky" profile. This means they might excel significantly in some areas while facing major challenges in others. For example, a client might have an encyclopedic knowledge of placental physiology (perhaps a deep dive into a special interest) but be completely unable to fill out the intake forms (executive dysfunction). They might be articulate and expressive but unable to process your verbal instructions about a prescription.

Noticing this discrepancy—the gap between high ability and significant struggle—is often the first clue that you might need to adapt your approach.

Look for sensory avoidance

How does your client interact with the room? Sensory input is often processed differently, and for many, it is magnified.

- **Light:** Are they wearing sunglasses indoors? Do they visibly flinch or squint under the fluorescent lights? Do they seem distracted by the glare off the floor?

- **Sound:** Do they cover their ears when a machine beeps or when there is loud talking nearby? Do they seem agitated by background noise that you tune out, like the ventilation system?

- **Touch:** Do they recoil from the cold gel of the ultrasound or the tightness of the blood pressure cuff? Are they constantly adjusting their clothing, perhaps bothered by tags or seams?

- **Scent:** Pregnancy heightens the sense of smell anyway, but look for extreme reactions to common clinical smells like hand sanitizer or cleaning products.

Communication styles that differ from the norm

Communication is not just about what is said. It is about how it is said, how information is received, and the unspoken social rules we often take for granted.

- **Literal Interpretation:** Many neurodivergent people interpret language very literally. If you say, "Hop up on the table," they might look confused. They are processing the word "hop." If you say, "This will just be a little pinch," and it hurts more than that, you have broken their trust. Avoid idioms, sarcasm, or vague language.

- **Bluntness or Directness:** Neurodivergent individuals often communicate very directly. They may skip the "small talk" and get straight to the point. This can sometimes be misinterpreted as rudeness, but it is usually just a preference for clear, unambiguous communication.

- **Difficulty with Open-Ended Questions:** Questions like "How are you feeling?" can be overwhelming. It is too broad. They may struggle to synthesize all the internal information and provide a concise answer.

- **Variations in Eye Contact:** Stop relying on eye contact as a measure of engagement. Many neurodivergent people find eye contact intensely uncomfortable or even painful. They might look away or close their eyes so they can focus better on what you are saying. Conversely, some might maintain intense eye contact because they have been taught to (masking), but you might notice it feels forced.

- **Processing Delays:** After you ask a question, there might be a pause. This does not mean they did not understand. It means they are processing. Get comfortable with silence. Do not rush to fill the space.

Executive function challenges in action

Executive function is the brain's management system—planning, organizing, prioritizing, and regulating emotions. Pregnancy places huge demands on executive function.

Cues in the clinic might include:

- Missing appointments or arriving very late (or extremely early) due to time blindness.

- Forgetting forms or necessary items.

- Difficulty filling out intake paperwork.

- Appearing overwhelmed by multi-step instructions (e.g., "Go to the lab, then schedule your ultrasound, and pick up this prescription").

Case example: Sarah's booking appointment

Sarah, 28, arrives for her first antenatal appointment. She is 10 minutes late and seems flustered, apologizing profusely. She is wearing large noise-canceling headphones and sunglasses. When the midwife, Maria, calls her name, Sarah does not respond until Maria walks over and gently touches her arm. Sarah jumps and pulls away sharply.

In the consultation room, Maria starts with the standard questions. When asked about her medical history, Sarah provides an extremely detailed, chronological account of every illness since childhood. She avoids eye contact, looking mostly at the floor. When Maria explains the upcoming appointments, Sarah just nods, but Maria notices Sarah is rhythmically tapping her fingers on her leg (stimming).

As the appointment concludes, Maria says, "Okay, so just pop down to the phlebotomist to get those labs done." Sarah freezes. She looks anxious. "Pop down? Where is it? Do I need a form? What do I say?"

*Analysis*

Maria recognizes several cues. The sensory gear (headphones, sunglasses) and the strong reaction to unexpected touch suggest sensory sensitivities. The detailed history and lack of eye contact are common communication styles. The stimming (finger tapping) suggests she might be self-regulating. Finally, the confusion over the vague instruction ("pop down") and the multi-step process indicate potential executive function challenges and literal interpretation.

Instead of labeling Sarah as anxious or difficult, Maria adapts. She dims the lights slightly. She slows down her speech. She provides a written, step-by-step list of the next actions, including a map to the phlebotomist and the exact words Sarah can use when she gets there.

**Navigating the conversation: How to sensitively inquire about sensory needs and communication preferences without demanding a diagnosis**

Okay, this is the tricky part. How do we ask about needs without asking, "So, do you have autism or something?" Demanding disclosure is invasive and can feel unsafe for the client. They may fear stigma, judgment, or even involvement from social services. And if they are undiagnosed, the question is pointless anyway.

Our goal is not to get a label. Our goal is to meet the access need.

The key is to normalize differences and focus on comfort and effective communication. We should be asking these questions of everyone, because, honestly, everyone benefits from individualized care.

## Focus on the environment not the person

Instead of asking what is "wrong" with them, ask what is "wrong" with the environment.

- "I know these lights are really bright. They bother me sometimes, too. Would it be helpful if I dimmed them?"

- "It can get noisy out in the hallway. Please let me know if you need a break or if any sounds are bothering you."

- "Some people find the texture of this gown scratchy. We have some softer ones if you prefer."

## Inquiring about communication preferences

Frame your questions around making sure **you** are communicating clearly.

- "I want to make sure I am explaining things in a way that works for you. Do you prefer information written down, visually, or by talking it through?"

- "We cover a lot in these appointments. What is the best way to help you process everything?"

- "Do you find it easier to communicate via email or text rather than phone calls? I know playing phone tag is the worst."

## Asking about processing and organization

Normalize the challenges of managing the logistics of pregnancy. It is a lot!

- "Pregnancy involves so many appointments. It is hard to keep track of. Do you use any specific tools like calendars or lists that we can help you with?"

- "When I give instructions, is it helpful if I break them down step-by-step or provide the big picture first?"

The magic question

If you are sensing distress or overwhelm, there is one question that often unlocks the necessary information:

**"What do you need to feel safe right now?"**

This question is open, non-judgmental, and centers the client's experience. They might say, "I need the lights off," "I need you to stop talking for a minute," or "I need to know exactly what is going to happen next."

## Supporting clients undergoing assessment or newly diagnosed during pregnancy

Pregnancy often triggers the recognition of neurodivergence. The massive life changes, the increased demands, and the intense sensory experiences can push coping strategies to their breaking point. Masking often becomes unsustainable. It is increasingly common for adults to seek assessment for autism or ADHD during the perinatal period.

This is an incredibly vulnerable time. A late diagnosis can bring a mix of emotions—relief, grief, anger, confusion. They are re-evaluating their entire lives through a new lens while simultaneously preparing for parenthood.

Validate and normalize their experience

The most important thing we can do is validate their feelings. They are not alone, and their struggles are real.

- Acknowledge the complexity: "It is a lot to process a new diagnosis while you are pregnant. Be gentle with yourself."

- Validate the relief and the grief: "It makes sense that you might feel relieved to have an explanation, but also sad about the support you needed and did not get."

- Normalize neurodivergence in parenthood: Reassure them that neurodivergent people are excellent parents. Their neurology brings unique strengths, such as attention to detail, creativity, and deep empathy.

Focus on immediate needs and adaptations

The diagnostic process can be long and stressful. Do not wait for the assessment to be complete before offering support.

- Implement adaptations now: If they suspect ADHD, offer strategies for organization and memory aids. If they suspect autism, address sensory needs and communication preferences right away.

- Help them advocate: Support them in communicating their needs to other providers, family members, and their workplace.

Connect them with community

Finding community with other neurodivergent adults is crucial. It combats isolation and provides a space to learn about neuro-affirming strategies.

- Encourage them to explore the neurodivergent community online (social media groups, blogs, organizations run by autistic adults or those with ADHD).

- Provide information on neurodiversity-affirming therapists or coaches. Be careful to avoid resources that focus on "curing" or masking.

Address fears about parenting

Many newly diagnosed adults worry about their ability to parent and fear judgment.

- Address the fear of stigma directly: Acknowledge that stigma exists but emphasize that a diagnosis does not define their capacity to parent.

- Focus on strengths: Help them identify how their neurodivergence can be a parenting superpower. For example, hyperfocus can lead to deep engagement in their child's interests.

## Documentation: Recording needs and preferences clearly and respectfully

Documentation is critical for continuity of care. It ensures that every member of the team understands the client's needs. However, documentation can also be a source of harm if done poorly. We must be mindful of the language we use.

Use strengths-based and neutral language

Avoid language that pathologizes or judges the client's behavior. Focus on what they need, not what is "wrong."

- **Instead of:** "Patient is uncooperative and refuses eye contact."

- **Write:** "Client prefers minimal eye contact for comfort during communication. Allow extra time for processing information."

- **Instead of:** "Patient is overly sensitive to noise and light."

- **Write:** "Client experiences sensory sensitivities. Minimize noise and use dim lighting when possible."

- **Instead of:** "Patient has poor organizational skills and missed last appointment."

- **Write:** "Client benefits from executive function support. Provide written appointment reminders (text preferred) and step-by-step instructions."

Focus on concrete adaptations

The documentation should clearly outline the specific adaptations that work.

- "Communication preferences: Prefers written information (email) over phone calls. Use clear, direct language. Avoid idioms."

- "Sensory needs: Provide noise-canceling headphones during procedures. Use a pediatric blood pressure cuff if possible due to tactile sensitivity."

Documenting diagnosis respectfully

If a client chooses to disclose a diagnosis, document it respectfully. However, be cautious about documenting suspected neurodivergence without the client's explicit consent.

- If the client discloses: "Client reports a diagnosis of autism (or ADHD)."

- If you suspect but the client has not disclosed: Focus purely on the access needs. Do not use diagnostic labels. For example, instead of "Appears autistic," write down the specific communication and sensory needs observed.

The importance of "Health Passports"

Encourage clients to create their own "Health Passport" or "About Me" document. This is written by the client and outlines their needs, preferences, and how best to support them. This can be added to their medical record.

This empowers the client and ensures their voice is centered. It can include things like: "I find it hard to process verbal information when stressed. Please write things down," or "I may rock or flap my hands when overwhelmed. This helps me regulate. I am still listening."

By documenting clearly and respectfully, we create a system that supports the client throughout their journey, no matter who they interact with.

---

**Key Takeaways from Chapter 4**

- Assume that a significant number of your clients may be undiagnosed or undisclosed neurodivergent, especially women and marginalized groups.

- Recognize the "spiky profile"—areas of high ability alongside significant challenges.

- Observe cues related to sensory avoidance (light, sound, touch), communication differences (literal interpretation, variations in eye contact), and executive function challenges (organization, time management).

- Inquire about needs sensitively by focusing on comfort and effective communication, rather than demanding a diagnosis. Ask, "What do you need to feel safe right now?"

- Support clients undergoing assessment by validating their experience, focusing on immediate needs, and connecting them with neuro-affirming resources.

- Documentation must be respectful, strengths-based, and focused on concrete adaptations, avoiding pathologizing language.

# Chapter 5: Adapting Antenatal Communication and Education

Effective communication is the foundation of safe and satisfying perinatal care. It is how we build trust, share information, and support informed decision-making. But here is the hard truth: the way we typically communicate in healthcare settings often fails neurodivergent clients. It is fast-paced, relies heavily on verbal instructions, and is full of jargon and abstract concepts.

For someone who processes information differently, needs extra time, or struggles with sensory overload, a standard antenatal appointment can be completely inaccessible. Research confirms this, showing that communication difficulties and not feeling understood are major barriers to healthcare for autistic adults (Doherty et al., 2022).

We cannot keep expecting our clients to adapt to our system. It is time for our system to adapt to our clients. This chapter is about the practical strategies for making antenatal communication and education truly neuro-affirming. It is about moving beyond just providing information to ensuring genuine understanding.

## Delivering information clearly: Avoiding jargon, using visual aids, and providing written summaries

The first step is simple: clean up our language. We are so immersed in medical terminology that we forget how confusing it is. And it is not just the big words. It is the vague phrasing, the idioms, and the assumptions we make.

Be direct and precise

Clarity is kindness. Use plain language and ditch the jargon. If you must use a medical term, explain it immediately.

- **Instead of:** "We need to monitor you for gestational hypertension."

- **Say:** "We need to keep a close eye on your blood pressure. Sometimes pregnancy causes high blood pressure, and we want to catch it early."

Be precise, especially when describing sensations. Keep in mind that many neurodivergent people interpret things literally.

- **Instead of:** "You might feel some discomfort."

- **Say:** "You will feel a sharp scratch when the needle goes in. It will last for about three seconds, and then it might feel achy for an hour."

The power of visual supports

Many neurodivergent individuals process information better when they can see it. Verbal information is transient—it disappears as soon as it is spoken. Visual information stays put.

Visual supports can include:

- **Diagrams and illustrations:** Use simple diagrams to explain physiological processes or procedures.

- **Checklists:** Provide checklists for symptoms to watch for, steps to take before a procedure, or items to pack in a hospital bag.

- **Visual schedules:** Use visual schedules to outline the agenda for the appointment or the timeline of pregnancy milestones.

When using visual aids, make sure they are clear and uncluttered. Avoid busy designs or distracting graphics.

Always provide written summaries

Look, everyone forgets most of what they hear in a medical appointment. This is especially true when stressed or experiencing sensory overload. Written summaries are non-negotiable.

These summaries should include:

- Key information discussed.
- Instructions for medications or treatments.
- Next steps and upcoming appointments.

The format matters. A dense block of text is overwhelming. Use bullet points, bold text, and lots of white space. Offer the summary in the client's preferred format—printed, emailed, or sent via the patient portal.

**The "Ask, Understand, Adapt" model**

Providing neuro-affirming care is not about following a script. It is about being flexible and responsive to the individual. The "Ask, Understand, Adapt" model is a simple framework for this process.

Step 1: Ask

We start by asking about the client's needs and preferences. We cannot assume we know what they need.

- **Ask about communication:** "How do you prefer to receive information?" "What is the best way for me to explain things clearly?"
- **Ask about sensory needs:** "Is the environment comfortable for you?" "Are there any sounds or lights that bother you?"
- **Ask about previous experiences:** "What has been helpful (or unhelpful) in previous healthcare interactions?"

Step 2: Understand

Once we have the information, we need to understand it within the context of the client's experience. This requires active listening and empathy.

- **Understand the "why":** If a client asks for the lights to be dimmed, understand that this is not a preference, but a genuine need to reduce sensory overload and anxiety.

- **Understand the impact of stress:** Recognize that stress can exacerbate sensory sensitivities and communication challenges.

- **Understand the spiky profile:** Keep in mind that a client may have areas of high ability and areas of significant struggle.

Step 3: Adapt

This is where we take action. We adapt our communication, the environment, and our processes.

- **Adapt communication:** Use clear language, provide visual aids, offer extra processing time.

- **Adapt the environment:** Dim the lights, reduce noise, offer sensory tools.

- **Adapt processes:** Offer flexible scheduling, streamline paperwork, provide predictable routines.

The "Ask, Understand, Adapt" model is a continuous loop. We keep asking, understanding, and adapting throughout the entire pregnancy journey.

Case example: Implementing "Ask, Understand, Adapt" with Tasha

Tasha is a 24-year-old pregnant client with diagnosed ADHD. She struggles with organization and time management and often misses appointments.

- **Ask:** The midwife asks Tasha what makes it difficult to attend appointments. Tasha explains that she often forgets the time (time blindness) and struggles with the multi-step process of getting ready and traveling to the clinic.

- **Understand:** The midwife understands that Tasha's challenges are related to executive dysfunction common in ADHD. It is not that she does not care; it is that the logistics are overwhelming.

- **Adapt:** The midwife implements several adaptations:

- o She sets up automated text message reminders 24 hours and 1 hour before each appointment.

- o She offers Tasha the first appointment of the day, so there is less waiting and a more predictable routine.

- o She helps Tasha create a visual checklist of the steps needed to get to the appointment.

- o She provides clear, written summaries highlighting the next steps.

By implementing these adaptations, Tasha attends her appointments consistently and feels more engaged in her care.

## Managing appointment anxiety: Predictability, clear agendas, and minimizing waiting times

Antenatal appointments can be a significant source of anxiety. The uncertainty, the sensory environment, and the social demands can all lead to overwhelm. One of the most effective ways to reduce this anxiety? Increase predictability.

For many autistic people and those with ADHD, the world can feel chaotic. Predictability provides a sense of safety and control (Advanced Autism Center, n.d.). When clients know what to expect, they can mentally prepare and regulate their nervous systems.

Minimize waiting times and communicate delays

Waiting rooms are often sensory nightmares. The uncertainty of how long the wait will be just adds to the anxiety.

- **Offer flexible scheduling:** Offer the first or last appointment of the day, which often have shorter waiting times.

- **Allow waiting in the car:** Offer the option for clients to wait in their car and receive a text message when you are ready.

- **Communicate delays proactively:** If you are running late, let the client know ASAP and provide a realistic estimate. Be honest. Do not say "five minutes" if it will be 30.

Provide clear agendas and structure

Knowing the structure of the appointment helps reduce uncertainty.

- **Outline the agenda at the beginning:** Start by briefly outlining what will happen. "Today we are going to check your blood pressure, listen to the baby's heartbeat, and talk about your ultrasound results."

- **Use visual schedules:** A simple visual checklist on a whiteboard can help the client track the progress of the appointment.

- **Signal transitions:** Give clear warnings before transitioning to a new activity. "Before we listen to the baby, I am going to put some cold gel on your belly."

Prepare for procedures and examinations

Physical examinations can be stressful due to the sensory input and vulnerability.

- **Explain the procedure step-by-step:** Describe exactly what you are going to do, what equipment you will use, and what it will feel like.

- **Use the "Tell-Show-Do" approach:** Show the equipment and demonstrate the procedure (if possible) before doing it.

- **Offer control and consent at every step:** Check in frequently. "Are you ready for me to start?" "Let me know if you need a break."

- **Allow for sensory supports:** Encourage the client to use sensory tools like fidget toys or noise-canceling headphones during the appointment.

By implementing these strategies, we can transform the antenatal appointment from a source of anxiety to a space of safety.

**Adapting parent education classes for sensory and social needs**

Traditional antenatal education classes? Often inaccessible. Think about it: a brightly lit room, crowded with strangers, hours of verbal instruction, and forced social interactions. It is a recipe for sensory overload and social anxiety.

We must rethink how we deliver this education.

Offer diverse formats and modalities

One size does not fit all. We need a range of options.

- **Online and self-paced options:** Online courses allow clients to learn in the comfort of their own home, control the sensory environment, and process information at their own pace.

- **One-on-one education:** Offer individualized sessions for clients who find group settings overwhelming.

- **Small group classes:** If group classes are offered, keep them small (no more than 5-6 couples) to reduce sensory and social demands.

Adapt the physical environment

If in-person classes are held, the environment must be managed.

- **Sensory-friendly setting:** Choose a location with natural lighting, minimal noise, and comfortable seating (think cushions or yoga balls, not just hard chairs).

- **Offer sensory tools:** Provide a basket of fidget toys, earplugs, and sunglasses.

- **Allow for movement:** Encourage participants to move around, stretch, or stim as needed. Normalize this by saying, "Please feel free to move your body in whatever way feels comfortable."

Adapt the content and delivery

The presentation style needs adaptation too.

- **Clear and structured content:** Break down information into small chunks. Use clear headings, bullet points, and visual aids.

- **Focus on practical skills:** Emphasize practical strategies rather than abstract concepts.

- **Provide written materials:** Offer detailed written materials to accompany the verbal instruction.

Manage social demands

The social aspect can be the hardest part.

- **No forced introductions or icebreakers:** These can be excruciating. If introductions are necessary, keep them brief and optional.

- **Structured social interactions:** If group activities are included, ensure they have a clear purpose and structure.

- **Respect communication differences:** Acknowledge and respect diverse communication styles. Normalize not making eye contact or needing extra time to respond.

Neuro-affirming content

The content of the classes should also be neuro-affirming.

- **Acknowledge sensory challenges:** Discuss strategies for managing sensory overload during labor, breastfeeding, and newborn care.

- **Address executive function:** Offer practical strategies for organization and prioritizing tasks in the postpartum period.

- **Normalize neurodivergent parenting:** Validate that there is no one "right" way to parent and that neurodivergent parents bring unique strengths.

By adapting our communication and education, we ensure that neurodivergent parents have the information and support they need to thrive. It requires intentional effort and a willingness to challenge the status quo, but the impact is immeasurable.

---

**Key Takeaways from Chapter 5**

- Deliver information clearly by using plain language, avoiding jargon, and being direct and precise.

- Use visual supports (diagrams, checklists) and always provide written summaries in an accessible format.

- Use the "Ask, Understand, Adapt" model: Ask about needs, understand the "why" behind them, and adapt your approach accordingly.

- Manage appointment anxiety by increasing predictability. Minimize waiting times, provide clear agendas, and prepare for procedures step-by-step.

- Adapt parent education classes for sensory and social needs. Offer diverse formats (online, one-on-one), create a sensory-friendly environment, and manage social demands respectfully.

# Chapter 6: The Neuro-Affirming Birth Plan

The birth plan. It is a standard part of antenatal care, often encouraged as a way for pregnant people to communicate their preferences. But let's be honest, the traditional birth plan often fails neurodivergent clients.

Standard templates focus mainly on medical interventions—epidural or no epidural, delayed cord clamping, skin-to-skin. Important, yes. But they completely overlook the fundamental access needs that make the difference between a traumatic birth and an empowering one for a neurodivergent person.

For someone with intense sensory sensitivities, the brightness of the operating room lights or the sound of the fetal monitor might be more distressing than the pain of contractions. For someone who struggles with verbal communication when stressed, the inability to advocate for themselves during labor can be terrifying.

We need to move beyond the standard template. We need to rethink the birth plan as an **Access Document**. It is not just a list of preferences; it is a tool for communication, accessibility, and self-advocacy. It is a way to ensure that the client's neurology is respected during one of the most vulnerable moments of their lives.

### Beyond the standard template: Creating a personalized "Access Document"

A personalized Access Document centers the client's lived experience and specific needs. It translates their neurology into concrete requests for adaptations in the birth environment.

Key components of an Access Document

Unlike a traditional birth plan, an Access Document prioritizes the following:

- **Communication protocols:** How the client communicates when stressed, and how the care team should communicate with them.

- **Sensory needs:** Specific sensory triggers and the adaptations needed to create a safe environment.

- **Coping mechanisms:** Strategies the client uses to self-regulate (e.g., stimming, movement) and how the care team can support them.

- **Executive function support:** Strategies for decision-making and managing uncertainty.

The process of creating the Access Document

This should be a collaborative process. It starts early in pregnancy and evolves.

- **Self-reflection:** Encourage the client to reflect on their sensitivities, preferences, and coping mechanisms. What makes them feel safe? What makes them feel overwhelmed?

- **Prioritization:** Help the client prioritize their needs. What are the non-negotiables?

- **Translation:** Translate the needs into clear, concise requests that the care team can easily understand and implement.

The format of the Access Document

The document must be easy to read for busy providers.

- **Keep it brief:** Ideally one page.

- **Use clear headings and bullet points.**

- **Use positive language:** Focus on what the client needs, rather than what they want to avoid. (e.g., "Please use a quiet voice" instead of "Do not talk loudly.")

- **Include a brief introduction:** A short paragraph explaining the purpose of the document and the client's neurology (if they choose to disclose).

**Example Introduction:**

"I am autistic (or have ADHD, sensory processing differences). This means my brain works differently, especially when I am stressed. This document outlines my access needs to ensure a safe and positive birth experience. Thank you for supporting me."

**Focusing on sensory needs, communication protocols, and coping mechanisms (e.g., stimming)**

Let's break down the key sections of the Access Document.

Sensory needs: Creating a sensory-safe environment

The birth environment is inherently intense. For a neurodivergent person, this intensity can lead to increased pain perception, anxiety, and shutdowns or meltdowns. The Access Document must clearly outline the specific adaptations needed.

- **Lighting:**
  - "Please keep the lighting dim. Use natural light or lamps if possible."
  - "I may wear an eye mask or sunglasses during labor."

- **Sound:**
  - "Please speak in a calm, quiet voice."
  - "Minimize unnecessary conversation and chatter."
  - "Please lower the volume of the fetal monitor if possible."

- **Touch:**
  - "Please ask for consent before touching me, including for exams or blood pressure checks."

- "Please describe what you are going to do before you do it."

- "I prefer deep pressure touch rather than light touch."

- **Smell:**

    - "Please avoid using strong scents (perfume, scented lotions)."

Communication protocols: Ensuring effective communication under stress

When stressed, neurodivergent individuals may struggle with verbal communication. They may find it difficult to process information or articulate their needs. The Access Document must detail how to communicate effectively.

- **Processing information:**

    - "Please use clear, direct language. Avoid jargon and idioms."

    - "Break down information into small steps."

    - "Allow me extra time to process information and respond. Please do not rush me."

- **Expressing needs:**

    - "If I am non-verbal or unable to speak, I will use [specific method, e.g., hand signals, communication cards, text-to-speech app]."

    - "If I seem distressed, please ask me simple, closed questions (yes/no)."

- **Interactions with the care team:**

    - "Please limit the number of people in the room."

    - "I may not make eye contact. This does not mean I am not listening."

Coping mechanisms: Supporting self-regulation

Neurodivergent individuals use various strategies to self-regulate. It is crucial that these are respected during labor.

- **Stimming:** Stimming (self-stimulatory behavior) involves repetitive movements or sounds that help regulate the nervous system (e.g., rocking, humming, flapping hands).

  - "I may stim during labor (e.g., rocking, humming). This helps me cope with pain and anxiety. Please do not interrupt me or ask me to stop."

  - "I will use specific sensory tools (e.g., fidget spinner, stress ball)."

- **Movement:**

  - "I need to be able to move freely. Please support intermittent monitoring if possible."

Case example: Excerpt from Maya's Access Document

Maya is autistic and has significant sensory sensitivities. Here is an excerpt from her Access Document:

**Introduction:** I am autistic. When I am in pain or overwhelmed, I may lose the ability to speak and become very sensitive to sensory input. Please support me by following these guidelines.

**Sensory Needs:**

- **Lighting:** Keep lights dim at all times.

- **Sound:** Speak softly. Minimize monitor volume. I will be wearing noise-canceling headphones.

- **Touch:** Ask consent before any touch. Describe sensations clearly (e.g., "cold gel," "sharp pinch").

**Communication:**

- Use clear, literal language.

- If I am non-verbal, I will use my communication cards (Yes/No/I need a break).

- Do not rush me for decisions. Give me time to process.

**Coping Mechanisms:**

- I will rock and hum during contractions. This is normal for me.

This document clearly outlines Maya's needs and provides concrete instructions for the care team.

## Planning for uncertainty: Using "If/Then" scenarios to manage anxiety about change

Birth is unpredictable. For neurodivergent individuals who rely on predictability to manage anxiety, this uncertainty can be terrifying. The fear of the unknown can lead to catastrophic thinking and increased distress (Sinha et al., 2014).

We can use "If/Then" scenarios to help clients plan for uncertainty and feel more prepared for unexpected changes. This strategy provides a structured way to think through possibilities and develop a plan.

The "If/Then" framework

The framework is simple: "If [unexpected event] happens, then [planned response]."

- **If** I need a Cesarean birth, **then** I want the lights in the OR dimmed if possible, and I want my partner to stay with me.

- **If** the baby needs to go to the NICU, **then** I want clear, written information about their condition.

- **If** my preferred midwife is not available, **then** I want the new midwife to read my Access Document before entering the room.

- **If** I feel overwhelmed and need a break, **then** I will use the hand signal for "stop," and the care team will pause and give me space.

Developing "If/Then" scenarios

Help the client identify their biggest fears. What are the "what ifs" that keep them up at night? Then, develop a concrete plan for responding.

- **Focus on what can be controlled:** We cannot control the outcome, but we can control the response. The scenarios should focus on adaptations that can be implemented even in unexpected situations.

- **Include sensory and communication needs:** Ensure that the planned responses include consideration for these needs. For example, if a transfer is needed, how can we manage the sensory environment during the transfer?

By using "If/Then" scenarios, we transform the unknown into something predictable. We give the client a roadmap for navigating uncertainty.

## Supporting executive function in decision-making (e.g., adapting the BRAIN framework)

Labor often requires making complex decisions under pressure. For neurodivergent individuals who struggle with executive function (planning, cognitive flexibility), this is incredibly challenging. Sensory overload and stress further impair their ability to process information and weigh options (Amen University, 2024).

We must adapt our approach to informed consent and decision-making.

The challenges of decision-making under stress

- **Difficulty processing complex information:** The influx of information about risks and benefits can be overwhelming.

- **Cognitive rigidity:** Difficulty considering different perspectives.

- **Emotional dysregulation:** Anxiety and fear can cloud judgment or lead to decision paralysis.

- **Time pressure:** The urgency of the situation exacerbates these challenges.

Adapting the BRAIN framework

The BRAIN framework (Benefits, Risks, Alternatives, Intuition, Nothing) is a common tool for decision-making. We can adapt it to better support executive function.

- **B - Benefits:** Explain the benefits clearly and concisely. Use visual aids.

- **R - Risks:** Explain the risks honestly, but avoid fear-mongering. Focus on the most common risks.

- **A - Alternatives:** Present the alternatives clearly. Limit the number of options if possible, as too many choices can be overwhelming.

- **I - Intuition:** Encourage the client to listen to their intuition, but acknowledge this can be difficult when stressed. Help them connect with their internal feelings.

- **N - Nothing (or Next):** What happens if we do nothing or wait? This is crucial for reducing time pressure.

Strategies for supporting executive function in decision-making

- **Break down the decision:** Break complex decisions into smaller steps.

- **Use visual aids:** Use decision trees or charts to illustrate the options.

- **Provide extra processing time:** Allow ample time. Do not rush them.

- **Minimize sensory input:** Reduce distractions to help the client focus.

- **Involve a support person:** Encourage the client to involve a trusted support person (partner, doula) in the decision-making process.

Case example: Decision-making during labor

A client with ADHD is in labor and considering an epidural. They are overwhelmed and unable to make a decision.

- **The adaptation:** The midwife recognizes the signs of executive function overload. She asks everyone else to leave the room to reduce sensory input. She sits down and calmly presents the information using a simple visual aid.

- **Breaking it down:** She breaks the decision into steps: "First, let's talk about the benefits. Then the risks. Then we can talk about other options."

- **Providing time:** She allows the client time to process each piece of information. She says, "Take your time. There is no rush."

By adapting her approach, the midwife supports the client's executive function and empowers them to make an informed decision that feels right for them.

The neuro-affirming Access Document is not a guarantee that everything will go perfectly. Birth is unpredictable. But it is a powerful tool for ensuring that the client's neurology is respected, their needs are accommodated, and their voice is heard during one of the most transformative moments of their lives.

---

**Key Takeaways from Chapter 6**

- Rethink the birth plan as a personalized "Access Document" that focuses on fundamental access needs.

- The Access Document should prioritize communication protocols, sensory needs, coping mechanisms (including stimming), and executive function support.

- Use clear, concise language and an accessible format (bullet points, headings).

- Use "If/Then" scenarios to plan for uncertainty and manage anxiety about change. Focus on what can be controlled (environment, communication) regardless of the clinical situation.

- Support executive function in decision-making by adapting the BRAIN framework, breaking down decisions, using visual aids, and providing extra processing time.

# Chapter 7: Creating the Autism and ADHD-Friendly Birth Environment

We talk a lot about the "vibe" of a birth space, don't we? We want it to feel calm, maybe even cozy. But look, for someone who is autistic or has ADHD, the environment isn't just about the vibe. It's not just a backdrop. It's an active participant in their experience. And honestly? The standard hospital environment is often the villain in the story.

Think about it. Hospitals are, by design, places of high sensory input. You've got the bright, buzzing fluorescent lights, the constant alarms, weird chemical smells, unfamiliar textures, and a revolving door of people you've never met. For a neurotypical brain—someone whose brain works in the typical way—this is stressful. But for a neurodivergent brain? It can be agonizing. Truly.

When a person is overloaded by sensory input, their ability to cope, communicate, and even process pain changes completely. They move into survival mode. Fight, flight, or freeze. And trust me, none of those are helpful when you are trying to have a baby. Sensory distress during labor isn't just unpleasant; it can actually interfere with the physiological process of birth and increase the risk of trauma (Hampton et al., 2022).

So, our job—our real job—is to turn down the sensory volume. We need to create a bubble of safety. A space where the birthing person can focus their energy on labor, not on managing the sound of the HVAC system rattling overhead. This isn't about being "extra." It's about basic accessibility. It's about making the space work for the person in the bed. And it starts long before the first contraction hits.

**The Sensory Audit A practical checklist**

You can't fix a problem until you know what it is. Right? This is where the sensory audit comes in. Now, that sounds formal, but it's really just a structured way of looking at a space and spotting potential sensory landmines.

Ideally, you do this during pregnancy. Maybe during a hospital tour or a specific meeting with the unit manager. If that's not possible, the birth partner or doula needs to do a quick audit as soon as you arrive. We need to look at every space the client might encounter: Triage, the labor ward, the operating theatre (yes, even if a surgical birth isn't planned), and the birth center.

**Triage is the first hurdle**

Triage. Oh, triage. It's often the worst part, sensory-wise. It's busy, loud, and unpredictable. You're usually sharing space or separated only by a thin curtain. The goal here is simple: survive the assessment and get moved to a more controlled environment as fast as possible.

What to look for in Triage:

- **Sound:** What alarms are constantly going off? How loud is the phone at the nurses' station? Can you hear conversations from other bays? Is there a loud TV blaring in the waiting area? (Why do they always do that?)

- **Light:** Are the main lights on? Are they fluorescent? (Almost certainly). Are there any seats facing away from the main lights?

- **Smell:** What hits you first? Strong cleaning products? Perfume from staff? Food smells?

- **Crowding:** How many people are milling around? How close are the bays? It can feel very exposed.

In triage, modifications are limited. The focus is on **defense**. This is the time to use the sensory toolkit immediately. Ear defenders, sunglasses, a hoodie pulled tight. The partner's job is to handle as much of the talking as possible. Let the birthing person conserve their energy.

**The labor ward offers more control**

Once you move to a labor room, you have more control. But standard hospital rooms still need work. When you get to the room, the audit needs to be quick and decisive.

What to look for in the Labor Ward:

- **Monitors and Alarms:** This is huge. Can the volume of the fetal heart rate monitor (CTG machine) be turned down or muted in the room? Often, the staff can still monitor the readouts at the central station. This is a critical modification to ask for.

- **Lighting:** Are there dimmer switches? If not, are there smaller side lamps we can use while turning off the main overhead lights? Can the blinds be fully closed?

- **The Bed and Linens:** Hospital linens are often stiff and scratchy. Can we swap them or layer home blankets on top?

- **The Bathroom:** How loud is the fan? Does the toilet flush aggressively? (I'm serious, these things matter when you're hyper-aware).

**Case Example Sarah's Room Setup**

Sarah is autistic and incredibly sensitive to light and sound. When she and her partner, Mark, got to the labor ward, Mark didn't even unpack the snacks first. He went straight into the sensory setup they had practiced. He turned off the main overhead fluorescent lights. Bingo. Then he plugged in two strings of battery-operated fairy lights they brought from home and draped them over the windowsill. He found the CTG machine and asked the midwife, "Sarah has severe sensory sensitivities. Can we please lower the volume on this machine significantly?" The midwife was happy to do it. Mark then placed Sarah's weighted blanket on the rocking chair. The room was instantly calmer. That quick setup stopped Sarah from becoming overwhelmed right at the start.

**The operating theatre is a sensory extreme**

If a Cesarean birth becomes necessary, the operating theatre (OT) presents a unique set of challenges. It is the most intense clinical environment possible. It's cold, bright, loud, and smells strongly of antiseptics. There are many people, and movement is restricted.

Auditing the OT in advance is tough, but knowing what to expect is key to preparation.

What to expect in the OT:

- **Brightness:** The surgical lights are incredibly bright and focused right where the action is.

- **Noise:** There is a lot of metallic clattering, suction noises (which can be very triggering), and multiple conversations happening at once.

- **Temperature:** OTs are kept cold. Request warm blankets for the chest and shoulders immediately.

- **Sensation:** The spinal block or epidural creates a profound lack of sensation in the lower body. This feeling of being disconnected from your own body can be very distressing in itself. Constant verbal reassurance and physical touch on the arms or face (where sensation remains) are crucial for grounding.

**The birth center is usually better but check anyway**

Birth centers are usually designed to be more home-like. They are often a better sensory fit. Softer lighting, less clinical equipment, quieter atmosphere. But don't assume it will be perfect.

What to look for in the Birth Center:

- **Water birth facilities:** The acoustics of a tiled room with a pool can be echoey. The sound of running water? Soothing for some, overwhelming for others.

- **Shared spaces:** Are the walls thin? Can you hear other people laboring?

- **Scents:** Do they use standard aromatherapy? If the client is sensitive to smells, this might be too much.

## Lighting Dimmers natural light eye masks

Let's talk about light. Visual input is often a major source of sensory overload. Fluorescent lighting, in particular, is the enemy. It's notoriously problematic for autistic and ADHD individuals.

Why? Because it flickers. Maybe you don't notice it, but the brain still registers it. It also often hums, and the quality of the light is harsh and clinical. Research has long linked fluorescent lighting to headaches, eye strain, and increased stress responses (Küller & Laike, 1998).

## Modifying the light we can control

The first step is always to maximize natural light during the day, if the client prefers it. Open the blinds. Natural light generally helps regulate the nervous system. But as night falls, or if the room is windowless (which, unfortunately, some are), we need alternatives.

Dimmer switches are the gold standard. If the room has them, use them. Keeping the lights low—think "cave-like" conditions—promotes relaxation. It supports the natural hormonal flow of labor. Oxytocin, the hormone needed for contractions, thrives in the dark.

If dimmers aren't available, we get creative.

1. **Turn off the overheads:** This is the simplest fix. Use side lamps, or the bathroom light with the door slightly ajar. Sometimes even the light from the medical equipment is enough if it's soft.

2. **Bring your own lighting:** I always recommend this. Battery-operated LED candles, fairy lights, or those little push lights can transform a clinical room into a sanctuary. They provide enough light for the medical staff to do their jobs but keep the overall atmosphere calm.

3. **Color:** Some neurodivergent individuals find certain colors regulating. Colored light filters or bulbs might be helpful, though this is getting into advanced setup.

## Defensive strategies when we cant change it

Sometimes we can't change the light source. In triage, during a medical assessment, or in the operating theatre, the lights will be bright. They have to be for safety. This is when defensive strategies are needed.

- **Eye masks:** A comfortable, well-fitting eye mask is essential for the hospital bag. It provides instant darkness and a sense of refuge. Some people prefer weighted eye masks for the added deep pressure.

- **Sunglasses:** Wearing sunglasses indoors might look unusual, but who cares? It is a highly effective way to reduce visual input. This is especially useful for clients who want to be aware of their surroundings but find the light painful.

- **Hats:** A baseball cap or a hat with a brim can reduce glare from overhead lights.

It's crucial that the medical team understands these are not fashion choices. These are accessibility aids. This should be clearly stated in the birth preferences document. "I wear sunglasses due to light sensitivity. This is not optional."

## Sound Reducing alarms minimizing chatter ear defenders preferred audio

Hospitals are noisy. There's no getting around it. Beep, beep, beep. It's the soundtrack of modern medicine. But the type of noise matters.

For many neurodivergent people, unexpected, sharp, or layered sounds are incredibly difficult to process.

Here's the thing: their brains often struggle to filter out background noise. That means everything is perceived at the same volume. The conversation at the nurses' station is just as loud as the person talking directly to them. It's exhausting and anxiety-provoking.

**Reducing unnecessary noise starting now**

The first line of attack is to reduce the noise at the source.

- **Alarms and Beeps:** As mentioned, the volume on monitoring equipment can often be turned down. Don't be afraid to ask. If an alarm sounds, the staff should explain what it means ("That's just the IV pump needing a new bag") and silence it quickly. Repetitive, unexplained alarms are a major trigger for anxiety.

- **Minimizing Chatter:** This is a big one, and sometimes the hardest to control. Medical staff often chat amongst themselves during labor. They might be discussing shift changes, weekend plans, or even other patients. This extraneous verbal input is incredibly distracting. We need to advocate for a "quiet room" policy. This means conversations should be directly related to the client's care and spoken in calm, low tones.

- **Doors and Foot Traffic:** The door to the room should remain closed. A sign on the door (e.g., "Quiet Please, Focusing on Birth. Knock softly and wait.") can remind staff to be mindful before entering. Minimize the number of people coming in and out.

**Case Example Alex's Auditory Overload**

Alex has ADHD and severe auditory processing issues. During their labor, the midwives were having a lively conversation in the corner of the room. It seemed harmless enough. But Alex found they couldn't focus on their breathing during contractions. They kept getting distracted by the midwives' words. Alex started to panic, their heart rate rising. The doula recognized the signs of auditory overload. She calmly approached the midwives and said, "Alex is having trouble filtering out conversation. Could we please keep the room quiet so they can focus?" The midwives immediately apologized and stopped talking. The difference in Alex's ability to cope with contractions was almost instant. It was that simple.

## Creating a preferred auditory environment

Once we've reduced the negative sounds, we can add positive auditory input. Sound can be a powerful tool for regulation and pain management.

- **Music:** Personalized playlists can be incredibly grounding. The music should be familiar and preferred by the client.

- **White, Brown, or Pink Noise:** Some individuals find a constant, low-level background noise soothing. It masks the sharper, unexpected sounds of the hospital. Brown noise, in particular, is often preferred by people with ADHD. A white noise machine or app can be very useful.

- **Affirmations:** Pre-recorded affirmations or guided meditations can help keep the client focused and calm.

- **The Human Voice:** A birth partner's calm, steady voice can be a lifeline. But remember, sometimes silence is golden. The client should dictate the level of verbal support they need. Don't assume they need constant coaching.

## Defensive tools for sound we cant control

When the environment is noisy and out of our control (like during a shift change or an emergency), defensive tools are necessary.

- **Ear Defenders:** These are the bulky headphones, like the ones used on a shooting range. They significantly reduce overall noise levels. Great for clients who want silence.

- **Noise-Canceling Headphones:** These actively counteract external sounds. They can be used with or without audio playing.

- **Earplugs:** Simple foam or silicone earplugs are a low-tech option. Loop earplugs, which reduce specific frequencies without blocking all sound, are often preferred by autistic individuals as they allow for communication while minimizing sensory stress.

## Touch and Texture The critical importance of explicit consent

Touch is perhaps the most intimate sense. During labor, it is highly charged. For neurodivergent individuals, touch can be soothing, grounding, or deeply distressing. It all depends on the type, the pressure, and, most importantly, whether it was expected and consented to.

## The consent imperative is non negotiable

I cannot stress this enough. I'm going to put it in bold so you really hear me: **Explicit consent is required for every single instance of touch.**

This includes medical procedures (like vaginal exams or placing monitors) but also comfort measures (like rubbing the back or holding a hand).

The standard medical practice of touching without explicit permission—assuming consent is implied—is deeply problematic for everyone. But it is particularly harmful to neurodivergent individuals who may have altered perceptions of touch or a history of trauma (which is, unfortunately, more common in this population) (Hughes et al., 2022).

We must establish a culture of consent from the very beginning.

1. **Ask First, Always:** The medical provider must ask, "Can I place the monitors on your belly now?" or "Would you like me to rub your back?"

2. **Wait for the Answer:** They must wait for a clear "yes" (verbal or non-verbal). Silence is not consent.

3. **Narrate the Action:** While performing the action, they should explain what they are doing. "I'm now touching your arm with the blood pressure cuff. It will feel tight."

If the client is non-verbal or unable to communicate clearly during labor, pre-agreed signals (like hand gestures or visual aids) must be used.

## Atypical responses to touch vary widely

We need to understand that responses to touch can vary widely. Don't assume what feels good.

- **Hypersensitivity (Tactile Defensiveness):** Light touch can be perceived as painful or irritating. Think about a scratchy tag on a shirt, but amplified tenfold. These clients may prefer deep pressure (like a firm squeeze on the shoulders) or no touch at all. Light stroking? Often a no-go.

- **Hyposensitivity (Sensory Seeking):** Some clients may crave intense tactile input. They might seek out strong hugs, use a weighted blanket, or press their bodies against hard surfaces. They need that input to feel grounded.

The key is to follow the client's lead. Ask. And then listen to the answer.

## Texture preferences matter too

The textures in the birth environment can have a significant impact on comfort and regulation.

- **Clothing:** Many neurodivergent individuals have strong preferences for clothing materials. Hospital gowns? They are often stiff, ill-fitting, and expose the body in ways that feel vulnerable. Clients should be encouraged to wear their own clothing if possible. Soft, seamless fabrics (like cotton or bamboo) are often preferred. Some might prefer tight clothing (compression), while others prefer loose, flowing garments.

- **Linens:** As mentioned, bringing familiar blankets and pillows from home can make a huge difference. The texture and smell of home linens provide a sense of safety.

- **Medical Equipment:** Things like blood pressure cuffs, electrode stickers, and ID bracelets can be irritating. The constant squeezing of the blood pressure cuff is a common trigger. Ask if the frequency of checks can be reduced if readings are stable.

## The power of positive touch

When consented to and preferred, touch can be a powerful tool. It can release oxytocin, reduce anxiety, and help the client feel grounded and supported.

- **Counter-pressure:** Firm pressure on the lower back during contractions can help alleviate pain.

- **Massage:** Deep pressure massage on the shoulders or feet can promote relaxation.

- **Hand Holding:** A simple hand squeeze can provide a vital connection.

But again, the client is in the driver's seat. What felt good five minutes ago might be irritating now. The birth team must be ready to adjust instantly.

## Smell Minimizing clinical odors

Smell is directly linked to the emotional centers of the brain. It's primal. And hospitals have a very distinct smell—a mix of antiseptics, cleaning products, and, well, other things. For those hypersensitive to olfactory input, this smell can be nauseating and anxiety-provoking.

Pregnancy itself often heightens the sense of smell. So a neurodivergent person who is pregnant is dealing with a double whammy of sensitivity.

## Reducing negative odors is the first step

Minimizing clinical odors is challenging in a hospital, but we can try.

- **Ventilation:** Opening a window (if possible and the air outside isn't worse) can help dissipate strong odors.

- **Unscented Products:** Requesting unscented soaps can be helpful. Staff should also avoid wearing strong perfumes or scented lotions.

- **Managing Triggers:** If the client is experiencing nausea, quickly removing sources of strong food odors or soiled linens is essential.

## Introducing preferred scents carefully

A more effective strategy is often to introduce preferred scents that can mask the clinical odors and provide comfort.

- **Aromatherapy:** Essential oils can be used, but with caution. Scent preferences are highly individual. What is calming for one person might be irritating for another. The client must choose the scents.

- **Application matters:** Instead of using a diffuser that fills the room (which can become overwhelming), apply a drop of essential oil to a cotton ball or a cloth. This way, it can be easily removed if it becomes too much.

- **Familiar Smells from Home:** The smell of a partner's t-shirt, a favorite blanket, or even a specific brand of soap can be incredibly comforting.

## A final word on environmental control

Creating a sensory-friendly birth environment is an ongoing process. It's not a "set it and forget it" situation. It requires constant vigilance, communication, and adaptation. The goal is not to create a perfect, silent bubble. Labor is messy. It's unpredictable.

The goal is to minimize **unnecessary** sensory stress. We want the client to focus their energy on the work of giving birth. When the environment supports the client's sensory needs, they are better able to stay regulated, manage pain, and participate actively in their care. It's about creating a space where they feel safe, respected, and empowered. And that, truly, is the foundation of a positive birth experience.

**Key Takeaways**

- The standard hospital environment can be overwhelming for autistic and ADHD individuals, potentially impacting the physiological process of labor.

- A sensory audit involves checking the birth spaces (Triage, Labor Ward, Theatre, Birth Centre) to identify and mitigate sensory triggers.

- Lighting should be adjustable. Favor dim, warm light over harsh fluorescents. Eye masks and sunglasses are essential defensive tools.

- Sound reduction means minimizing alarms and chatter. Preferred audio (music, white noise) and ear defenders can help manage auditory input.

- Explicit consent is mandatory for all touch. Every single time.

- Understanding the client's preference for deep pressure vs. light touch is crucial.

- Familiar textures (clothing, linens from home) provide comfort and regulation.

- Minimizing clinical odors and introducing preferred scents cautiously can help manage olfactory sensitivities.

# Chapter 8: Supporting the Neurodivergent Client in Labor

Okay, so we've set the stage. We've modified the environment. The lights are dimmed, the noise is minimized, and we've established the ground rules about consent. Now, the real work begins. Labor.

Labor is intense. It's unpredictable. It's demanding for anyone. But for the autistic or ADHD client, the experience is often amplified. They are navigating the physical demands of labor while simultaneously managing their unique sensory processing, communication styles, and emotional regulation needs. It's a lot.

Supporting a neurodivergent client in labor requires a shift in perspective. We can't rely on assumptions about how labor "should" look or feel. We have to throw out the standard playbook. Seriously, toss it out. We need to tune in to the individual right in front of us. This means understanding how they experience pain, recognizing their self-regulatory behaviors (even if they look unusual), adapting how we talk to them, and minimizing unnecessary interruptions.

This isn't just about being "nice." It's about providing safe, effective, and affirming care.

**Atypical responses to pain**

Pain is a universal experience during labor. But how that pain is perceived and expressed? That varies dramatically among neurodivergent individuals. The standard pain scale—you know, the "rate your pain from 1 to 10" thing—is often completely useless here.

Why? It comes down to differences in sensory processing and **interoception**. Interoception is your ability to sense the internal state of your body. It's how you know you're hungry, thirsty, or in pain. Many neurodivergent people have differences in interoception

(DuBois et al., 2016). This leads to two main possibilities: extreme sensitivity or under-responsiveness.

**Hypersensitivity to pain means extreme sensitivity**

Many autistic and ADHD individuals are hypersensitive to sensory input. And yes, this includes pain. What might be perceived as mild discomfort by a neurotypical person can be experienced as excruciating, overwhelming pain by someone who is hypersensitive.

These clients may exhibit intense reactions to contractions early in labor. They might become highly distressed, anxious, or unable to cope long before they reach active labor. It's very easy for medical providers to dismiss this. They might think the client is being "dramatic" or has a low pain threshold. But this is a misunderstanding of their neurology. The pain is real. It is overwhelming their nervous system.

Supporting the hypersensitive client involves:

1. **Validation:** Acknowledge that their pain is real and intense. Never minimize their experience. Saying "It's just early labor" is not helpful.

2. **Early Access to Pain Relief:** Discussing pain relief options (both medication and non-pharmacological methods like water immersion) early. Make sure they are readily available.

3. **Sensory Modulation:** Reducing other sensory inputs (light, sound) to help the nervous system cope with the pain input. Turn down the noise so they can focus on the contractions.

4. **Grounding Techniques:** Using deep pressure, weighted blankets, or focused breathing to help regulate the nervous system.

**Hyposensitivity to pain means under responsiveness**

On the other end of the spectrum, some neurodivergent individuals are hyposensitive to pain. They may not register pain until it is extremely severe. This is often linked to those difficulties with interoception we talked about. They might not notice the early signs of labor or realize how far along they are.

These clients might appear calm, quiet, and even detached during labor. They might be chatting or scrolling on their phone despite having strong contractions. This can lead to tricky situations. Like very fast labors (precipitous birth) or unrecognized complications.

Supporting the hyposensitive client involves:

1. **Objective Monitoring:** Relying on objective signs of labor progress (like contraction frequency and duration, or cervical dilation) rather than the client's self-reported pain levels.

2. **Scheduled Check-ins:** Regularly asking the client to tune into their body. "What sensations are you feeling right now?"

3. **Visual Aids:** Using visual timers or diagrams to help the client understand the progression of labor.

## The pain and anxiety spiral

Another complicating factor is the interplay between pain and anxiety. For neurodivergent individuals, anxiety about the unknown, loss of control, or sensory overload can amplify the perception of pain. The increased pain then leads to more anxiety. It's a vicious cycle.

Breaking this cycle requires addressing both the pain and the underlying anxiety. This means providing clear information, maintaining a calm environment, and offering consistent reassurance.

## Case Example Maria's Silent Labor

Maria is autistic and hyposensitive to pain. She arrived at the hospital only because her water had broken. She reported feeling only mild discomfort. She was chatting quietly with her partner, seemingly relaxed. The midwife assumed she was in early labor and left them alone. Which makes sense, right? But an hour later, Maria suddenly started making low grunting noises and said she felt "pressure." The midwife checked her and found she was fully dilated. The baby was coming. Maria had gone through transition—the most intense phase of labor—without showing any outward signs of distress. The medical team was scrambling. This situation could have been avoided if the team had relied on objective monitoring rather than Maria's subjective report of pain.

**Recognizing and supporting stimming during contractions**

Stimming (self-regulatory behaviors) is a key coping mechanism for many autistic and some ADHD individuals. Stimming involves repetitive movements, sounds, or manipulation of objects.

Why do people stim? It serves several important functions. It helps regulate the nervous system, express emotions, manage sensory overload, and cope with pain (Kapp et al., 2019).

During labor, stimming might look different than usual. It might become more intense, more frequent, or change in form. Common examples of stimming during labor include:

- **Rocking or Swaying:** Rhythmic movement is often soothing and helps manage the rhythm of contractions.

- **Hand Flapping or Clapping:** This can be an expression of excitement, anxiety, or pain.

- **Vocalization:** Humming, singing, chanting, or repeating specific words or phrases (this is called echolalia).

- **Tapping or Drumming:** Rhythmic tapping on the bed, the wall, or their own body.

- **Object Manipulation:** Squeezing a stress ball, rubbing a smooth stone, or twisting a piece of fabric.

**Stimming is not a problem to be solved**

This is the most important thing to understand: Stimming is a healthy and necessary behavior. It is **not** something to be stopped or discouraged. In fact, suppressing stimming can lead to increased distress, anxiety, and even meltdowns or shutdowns.

When a client is stimming during labor, it means they are actively working to cope with the intensity of the experience. It is a sign that their self-regulatory mechanisms are working.

## How to support stimming

The role of the birth team is to recognize, respect, and support stimming.

1. **Do Not Interfere:** Never try to stop the client from stimming. Do not hold their hands, ask them to be quiet, or tell them to "just relax." (Telling anyone in labor to relax is generally bad advice, anyway).

2. **Provide Space and Safety:** Ensure the client has enough space to move freely and safely. If they are rocking vigorously, make sure they won't hurt themselves.

3. **Offer Stimming Tools:** Make sure the client has access to their preferred stimming tools (e.g., stress balls, textured fabrics).

4. **Incorporate Stimming into Coping:** Stimming can be integrated into pain management. For example, rhythmic rocking can be synchronized with breathing during contractions.

5. **Educate the Medical Team:** Ensure that the medical staff understands what stimming is and why it is important. This should be clearly noted in the birth preferences.

## Case Example Ben's Vocalizations

Ben is autistic and uses vocal stimming (making sounds) to cope with stress. During his contractions, he would make a loud, repetitive humming sound. It was deep and rhythmic. One of the nurses, trying to be helpful, kept asking him to "take a deep breath" instead of humming. Ben became increasingly agitated. He started hitting his head with his hands—a clear sign of distress. His doula intervened. She explained to the nurse that the humming *was* his way of breathing and coping. She encouraged Ben to hum as loudly as he needed. Once the nurse stopped interfering, Ben was able to find his rhythm again and the distress behaviors stopped.

## Communication during active labor

Communication is challenging enough during active labor. The birthing person is focused inward, riding the waves of contractions. The ability to process complex language goes way down. For the neurodivergent client, these challenges are magnified.

Autistic individuals may have difficulties with receptive language (understanding what is being said) and expressive language (communicating their needs) when under stress. ADHD individuals may struggle with attention, working memory, and filtering out distractions.

So, how do we communicate effectively when the pressure is on?

### Keep it short clear and concrete

Forget about long explanations, abstract concepts, or nuanced language. Communication needs to be direct, concise, and focused on the immediate situation.

- **Use Short Sentences:** Instead of saying, "We are going to move you to a different position now because it might help the baby rotate and make your contractions more effective," just say, "Let's turn on your side."

- **Use Concrete Language:** Avoid metaphors or euphemisms. Be specific about what is happening and what needs to be done.

- **Speak Slowly and Calmly:** A calm, steady voice is easier to process than a rushed, high-pitched one.

- **Allow Processing Time:** This is key. After asking a question or giving an instruction, pause. Wait for a response. Neurodivergent individuals often need extra time to process information, especially when stressed. Do not rush them or repeat the question immediately. Just wait.

## Minimize verbal input during contractions

During a contraction, the client is completely focused on managing the pain. Any verbal input at this time can be distracting and overwhelming. It can pull them out of their focus. Save conversations and instructions for the breaks between contractions.

## Use pre agreed keywords or non verbal aids

This is where prenatal preparation is crucial. During pregnancy, work with the client to establish communication strategies for labor.

- **Keywords:** Agree on specific keywords that have clear meanings. For example, "Red" could mean "Stop immediately," "Yellow" could mean "I need a break," and "Water" could mean "I want to get in the tub."

- **Non-verbal Signals:** Establish hand signals for "yes," "no," and "I don't know." Thumbs up/thumbs down works well.

- **Visual Aids:** Use visual aids (like picture cards or diagrams) to communicate information and choices. Showing a picture of different labor positions can be much easier than describing them verbally.

## The role of the advocate

The birth partner or doula plays a crucial role in facilitating communication. They can act as an interpreter. They translate the medical jargon into language the client understands, and communicate the client's needs to the medical team.

They should also handle as much of the external communication as possible (like answering questions from the staff). This allows the client to stay focused and conserve energy.

## Understanding non speaking periods

It is common for autistic individuals to lose the ability to speak when overwhelmed or in intense pain. This is sometimes called situational mutism or going non-speaking. It is not a conscious choice. It is a neurological response to stress.

If the client becomes non-speaking, do not panic. Do not force them to talk. Switch to non-verbal communication strategies (visual aids, hand signals). Ensure the medical team understands this is a possibility and knows how to respond. Crucially, being non-speaking does not mean they cannot understand what is being said to them.

## Monitoring and assessments Bundling care

Continuous monitoring and assessments are a standard part of hospital birth. They are necessary to ensure safety. But let's be real: they can also be incredibly disruptive and distressing for the neurodivergent client.

Every time a provider enters the room, performs a procedure, or asks a question, it interrupts the client's focus. It increases sensory input. It can trigger anxiety. For someone struggling to stay regulated, these constant interruptions can be devastating.

## Minimizing interruptions is the goal

The goal is to minimize the frequency and intensity of interruptions while still ensuring safe care.

- **Bundling Care:** This is a simple but effective strategy. Instead of performing assessments one at a time (checking blood pressure now, then temperature 15 minutes later, then adjusting the monitors 10 minutes after that), bundle them together. Perform all necessary assessments at once, and then leave the client alone for a period of time.

- **Informed Consent for All Procedures:** As discussed in Chapter 7, explicit consent is required for all procedures. This includes monitoring. The provider should explain what they are going to do, why it is necessary, and ask for permission before proceeding.

- **Minimizing Vaginal Exams:** Vaginal exams are particularly invasive and distressing for many neurodivergent individuals, especially those with a history of trauma or tactile sensitivity. They should be kept to a minimum, performed only when necessary, and done with extreme sensitivity and consent.

## Wireless monitoring options are a game changer

The standard method of fetal monitoring involves elastic belts strapped tightly around the abdomen, connected by wires to a machine. This can be incredibly uncomfortable and restrictive for someone with tactile sensitivities. It also limits movement, which is essential for coping with labor pain and supporting progress.

Wireless monitoring (telemetry) is a game-changer. It allows the client to move freely, use the tub or shower, and find comfortable positions, all while continuously monitoring the baby's heart rate.

If wireless monitoring is available, advocate strongly for its use. It can significantly improve the sensory experience of labor and support the client's autonomy.

## Creating a predictable rhythm

Predictability is often key to managing anxiety for neurodivergent individuals. While labor itself is unpredictable (that's the nature of the beast), we can create a predictable rhythm for monitoring and assessments.

- **Explain the Schedule:** Inform the client about the expected frequency of assessments (e.g., "We will check your blood pressure every hour").

- **Give Warnings:** Before entering the room or starting a procedure, give a clear warning. (e.g., Knocking on the door and saying, "We are coming in now to check the baby's heart rate").

## The importance of rest and recovery

Labor is a marathon, not a sprint. Rest is essential. By minimizing interruptions and creating a calm environment, we support the client's ability to rest and recover between contractions. This conserves energy and helps maintain emotional regulation.

**Embracing the journey**

Supporting a neurodivergent client in labor is a delicate dance. It requires deep listening, keen observation, and a willingness to adapt our approach constantly. There is no one-size-fits-all solution.

When we honor the client's unique needs, validate their experience of pain, support their self-regulatory behaviors, and communicate with clarity and respect, we create a space where they can access their inner strength. We help them navigate the intensity of labor in a way that feels safe, affirming, and empowering.

---

**Key Takeaways**

- Neurodivergent individuals may experience pain differently, showing extreme sensitivity (hypersensitivity) or under-responsiveness (hyposensitivity). Standard pain scales are often ineffective.

- Stimming (self-regulatory behaviors) is a healthy coping mechanism during labor. It should be recognized, respected, and supported, never suppressed.

- Communication during active labor must be short, clear, and concrete. Use pre-agreed keywords, non-verbal aids, and allow extra processing time.

- Be prepared for the possibility of the client becoming non-speaking (situational mutism) under stress.

- Minimize interruptions by bundling care (performing multiple assessments at once).

- Wireless monitoring options improve comfort, support movement, and reduce sensory distress.

# Chapter 9: Navigating Interventions and Emergencies

We all hope for a smooth, straightforward birth. We prepare, we plan, we create a supportive environment. But birth is inherently unpredictable. Sometimes, interventions become necessary. Sometimes, emergencies happen. These situations are stressful for everyone involved. But for the autistic or ADHD client? The stress is magnified tenfold.

When things go off-script, the sensory overload increases dramatically. The pace quickens, the noise level rises, the number of people in the room multiplies. The sense of control, which is so crucial for neurodivergent individuals, evaporates. This rapid escalation can trigger extreme anxiety, panic, meltdowns, or shutdowns.

Navigating interventions and emergencies requires a delicate balance. We need to provide urgent medical care while maintaining a supportive, affirming environment. It requires clear communication, specialized consent processes, and a deep understanding of the client's unique needs. Our goal is to ensure that even in high-stress situations, the client feels safe, respected, and informed. We want to prevent trauma, not just ensure survival.

## Maintaining an affirming environment during high stress situations

When an intervention or emergency occurs, the focus naturally shifts to the medical tasks at hand. The physiological safety of the birthing person and the baby is the priority. Absolutely. But that doesn't mean that psychological safety goes out the window. In fact, it becomes even more critical.

A distressed, panicked client cannot participate in their care. They cannot process information or make decisions. Furthermore, the trauma associated with a poorly managed emergency can have long-lasting effects on mental health and bonding (Reed et al., 2017).

### The power of calm presence

The demeanor of the birth team is contagious. If the staff is calm, confident, and communicative, it helps regulate the client's nervous system. If the staff is rushed, panicked, or shouting, it escalates the situation. It's as simple as that.

Even in an emergency, medical providers must strive to maintain a calm presence. This means:

- **Lowering the Volume:** Speaking in calm, low tones. Avoiding shouting or alarms unless absolutely necessary.

- **Moving Deliberately:** Moving quickly but deliberately. Avoiding rushed or chaotic movements.

- **Minimizing Chatter:** Keeping conversations focused on the immediate tasks. No side conversations.

### The role of the anchor

The birth partner or doula plays a vital role as an "anchor" during high-stress situations. They provide a familiar, trusted presence in a sea of strangers.

The anchor's job is to:

1. **Stay Close:** Staying physically close to the client, maintaining eye contact (if preferred), and offering consented touch (like holding a hand or placing a hand firmly on the shoulder).

2. **Provide Reassurance:** Offering constant verbal reassurance in simple, clear language. ("I am here with you." "You are safe.")

3. **Facilitate Communication:** Acting as a liaison between the medical team and the client, explaining what is happening and communicating the client's needs.

## Sensory mitigation in crisis

While the overall sensory input increases during an emergency, we can still take steps to mitigate the distress.

- **Defensive Tools:** Offering ear defenders or an eye mask if the client is overwhelmed by the noise and light.

- **Grounding:** Using deep pressure or a weighted blanket (if practical) to help the client feel grounded.

- **Focusing Attention:** Directing the client's attention to a specific object or voice to help filter out the chaos.

## Case Example The Emergency Transfer

Jamie has ADHD and a history of trauma. During their labor at a birth center, the baby's heart rate started dropping significantly. An emergency transfer to the hospital was initiated. The paramedics arrived quickly. The sirens were blaring, and everyone was rushing. Jamie started screaming and trying to get out of the stretcher. They were having a full-blown meltdown. The doula recognized this not as defiance, but as a response to the sensory overload and loss of control. She placed her hands firmly on Jamie's shoulders (a pre-agreed grounding technique) and said calmly, "Jamie, I am here. We are moving to the hospital to keep you and the baby safe." She then asked the paramedic if the siren could be turned off once they were on the main road. This simple intervention helped Jamie regulate enough to cope with the transfer.

## Communication protocols during emergencies

In an emergency, clear, efficient communication is essential. But the standard medical communication style—rapid-fire, jargon-heavy, multiple overlapping conversations—is completely inaccessible to a neurodivergent person under stress.

We need established communication protocols for emergencies. Protocols that prioritize clarity, conciseness, and respect.

## The designated communicator

One of the most effective strategies is to designate a **single person** to communicate with the client. This should ideally be someone the client knows and trusts (like their primary midwife or obstetrician). If that's not possible, it should be the most senior person in the room.

This designated communicator is the only one who speaks directly to the client. Everyone else in the room communicates through them or amongst themselves quietly. This minimizes the overwhelming effect of multiple voices and conflicting information.

## The how of communication

How information is communicated is just as important as what is being said.

1. **Use the Client's Name:** Start every communication by using the client's name to get their attention.

2. **Be Direct and Honest:** Explain what is happening in simple, clear language. Avoid jargon and euphemisms. Be honest about the situation without being alarmist.

3. **Give Clear Instructions:** If the client needs to do something, give clear, step-by-step instructions. (e.g., "Jamie, I need you to turn on your side now.")

4. **Provide Regular Updates:** Even if nothing has changed, provide regular updates. Silence can be terrifying.

## The What Why How Framework

A useful framework for communicating during interventions is the "What, Why, How" approach. It provides a clear, logical structure for information, making it easier to process.

- **What:** What is happening? (e.g., "The baby's heart rate is low.")

- **Why:** Why is this a concern? (e.g., "It means the baby might not be getting enough oxygen.")
- **How:** What are we going to do about it? (e.g., "We are going to give you oxygen and move you to the operating room for a Cesarean birth.")

## The sensory experience of the operating theatre

If a Cesarean birth becomes necessary, the client will be moved to the operating theatre (OT). As we discussed in Chapter 7, the OT is a sensory nightmare. It is the most intense clinical environment possible. Understanding the sensory experience of the OT is key to preparing and supporting the client.

## The sensory assault

Let's break down the sensory assault of the OT. It's important to know what's coming.

- **Visual:** Incredibly bright overhead lights, metallic surfaces, multiple people in scrubs, unfamiliar equipment.
- **Auditory:** Loud noises, clattering instruments, suction sounds, alarms, multiple conversations.
- **Tactile:** Cold temperature, hard operating table, restrictive movement (arms might be strapped down, though this should be avoided if possible), strange sensations during the surgery (like pressure, tugging).
- **Olfactory:** Strong smells of antiseptics and sterilization chemicals.
- **Interoceptive:** The profound lack of sensation due to the anesthesia can be deeply distressing. The feeling of being disconnected from the lower half of the body can trigger panic and dissociation.

## Mitigating the sensory overload in the OT

While we cannot change the fundamental nature of the OT, we can take steps to mitigate the sensory overload and support the client's comfort.

- **Preparation:** If time allows, explain to the client what to expect in the OT, focusing on the sensory aspects.

- **Music/Audio:** Playing preferred music or audio through earphones (usually one earbud is allowed) can provide a familiar auditory anchor and mask the distressing sounds of the OT.

- **Visual Modifications:** Offering an eye mask or sunglasses before the surgery begins. Lowering the drape slightly (if possible) so the client can see their partner.

- **Temperature Control:** Asking for warm blankets on the chest and shoulders. Constantly checking if they are warm enough.

- **Grounding Touch:** The partner or doula providing constant physical touch on the arms, face, or shoulders (where sensation remains).

- **Narrating the Experience:** The anesthesiologist or designated communicator explaining the sensations the client might feel. "You might feel some pressure now." "You will feel some tugging."

- 

## Supporting connection and bonding

A Cesarean birth is still a birth. We must strive to create a space where the client feels connected to the experience and can bond with their baby.

- **Immediate Skin-to-Skin:** Facilitating immediate skin-to-skin contact in the OT, if safe and practical. This helps regulate the baby and the parent (Moore et al., 2016).

- **Respecting the Moment:** Minimizing chatter and creating a calm atmosphere during the moment of birth.

## Informed Consent Ensuring genuine understanding when time is limited

Informed consent is a fundamental human right. It means the client must be given clear information about the proposed procedure, the risks and benefits, and the alternatives. And they must voluntarily agree to it.

However, obtaining genuine informed consent during an emergency is incredibly challenging. The client is stressed, in pain, and possibly overwhelmed. Their ability to process complex information and make decisions is significantly impaired. For neurodivergent individuals, who often need extra processing time and struggle with communication under stress, this challenge is even greater.

### The problem with standard consent processes

The standard medical consent process—quickly explaining the procedure and asking the client to sign a form—is often inadequate in emergencies. It prioritizes liability protection over genuine understanding. Let's be clear: A signature on a form does not equal informed consent.

### Strategies for enhanced informed consent

We need strategies to enhance the informed consent process, even when time is limited.

1. **Prenatal Discussions:** The foundation of informed consent is laid during pregnancy. Discussing potential interventions and emergencies (like Cesarean birth, episiotomy, or instrumental delivery) in advance, when the client is calm and can process information, is crucial. Document these preferences clearly in the birth plan.

2. **Simple, Clear Language:** Use simple, clear language and avoid jargon. Use the "What, Why, How" framework.

3. **Visual Aids:** Using visual aids (like diagrams or infographics) to explain the procedure can enhance understanding, if time allows.

4. **Check for Understanding:** After explaining the procedure, ask the client to repeat back what they understood. ("Can you tell me what we are planning to do?")

5. **Allow Processing Time (Even if Brief):** Even in an emergency, there is usually time for a brief pause. A 30-second pause to allow the client to process the information and ask questions can make a huge difference.

6. **The Role of the Advocate:** The birth partner or doula can help facilitate the consent process by asking clarifying questions and ensuring the client's voice is heard.

### Consent in true emergencies

In a true life-threatening emergency (like massive hemorrhage or placental abruption), there may not be time for a full informed consent process. Medical providers are ethically and legally obligated to act to save the client's life.

However, even in these situations, communication remains essential. The providers should still explain what they are doing and why. And as soon as the situation stabilizes, a full debriefing must occur.

### Differentiating between a meltdown/shutdown and an obstetric emergency

This is perhaps the most critical and challenging aspect of caring for neurodivergent clients during labor. How do we distinguish between a response to sensory overload or emotional distress (like a meltdown or shutdown) and a genuine obstetric emergency?

Misinterpreting a meltdown as a medical crisis can lead to unnecessary interventions and trauma. Conversely, misinterpreting a medical crisis as a meltdown can have devastating consequences.

**Understanding meltdowns and shutdowns**

- **Meltdown:** A meltdown is an externalized response to overwhelm. It might involve crying, screaming, shouting, kicking, hitting, or other intense behaviors. It is not a tantrum. It is a complete loss of behavioral control due to sensory or emotional overload.

- **Shutdown:** A shutdown is an internalized response to overwhelm. It might involve becoming withdrawn, unresponsive, non-speaking, or seemingly detached. The client might appear calm on the surface, but internally they are in crisis.

**Key differentiating factors**

Differentiating between these requires a holistic assessment. We must look at both physiological and behavioral signs.

1. **Physiological Signs:** Obstetric emergencies are usually accompanied by specific physiological signs. Changes in vital signs, abnormal fetal heart rate, bleeding. Meltdowns and shutdowns typically do not cause these physiological changes (although heart rate and blood pressure might increase due to stress).

2. **Triggers:** Meltdowns and shutdowns are usually triggered by specific sensory or emotional events. Increased noise, unexpected touch, loss of control. Obstetric emergencies can occur without any obvious external trigger.

3. **Response to Intervention:** Meltdowns and shutdowns often improve with sensory mitigation and emotional support. Reducing noise, providing grounding touch. Obstetric emergencies require specific medical interventions.

## The importance of baseline knowledge

Knowing the client's baseline behavior and typical responses to stress is essential. This information should be gathered during prenatal care and communicated to the medical team. "When I am overwhelmed, I stop talking and rock back and forth."

## The when in doubt protocol

When in doubt, the priority is always to rule out an obstetric emergency first. Perform the necessary medical assessments (check vital signs, fetal heart rate, etc.).

However, these assessments must be done in a way that minimizes further distress. Explain what you are doing, ask for consent, and maintain a calm demeanor.

If the medical assessment is normal, then the focus should shift to addressing the underlying sensory or emotional distress.

## Case Example The Postpartum Hemorrhage Scare

Avery is autistic. Shortly after giving birth, they started shaking uncontrollably, crying, and repeating the phrase "too much, too much." The nurse thought they might be having a seizure or a postpartum hemorrhage (severe bleeding). She called for help. Suddenly the room was full of people. Avery became even more distressed. The midwife, who knew Avery well, recognized this as a meltdown. It was triggered by the intensity of the birth and the sudden increase in sensory input. She quickly cleared the room, dimmed the lights, and placed a weighted blanket on Avery's chest. She also checked Avery's bleeding and uterus, which were normal. With the sensory mitigation and calm support, Avery gradually calmed down. Crisis averted.

## A final reflection on crisis management

Navigating interventions and emergencies with neurodivergent clients is challenging. No doubt about it. It requires a fundamental shift in how we approach crisis management in the birth space. It requires us to prioritize communication, consent, and psychological safety alongside physiological safety.

When we do this well, we not only ensure the best possible medical outcomes, but we also minimize the risk of trauma and support the client's long-term well-being. We affirm their dignity, respect their autonomy, and honor their unique needs, even when the pressure is on.

---

**Key Takeaways**

- Interventions and emergencies are highly stressful for neurodivergent clients due to increased sensory overload and loss of control.

- Maintaining a calm presence, providing an anchor (a trusted support person), and mitigating sensory distress are crucial during high-stress situations.

- Communication protocols should include a designated communicator who speaks clearly, calmly, and honestly, using the "What, Why, How" framework.

- The operating theatre presents significant sensory challenges. Mitigation strategies include preferred audio, temperature control, grounding touch, and narration of the experience.

- Informed consent requires genuine understanding, even when time is limited. Use simple language, check for understanding, and rely on prenatal discussions.

- Differentiating between a meltdown/shutdown and an obstetric emergency requires a holistic assessment, considering physiological signs, triggers, and response to intervention.

# Chapter 10: The Immediate Postpartum Period and the Ward

You did it. The baby is here. Whether the birth went exactly as planned (does it ever?) or took a completely unexpected turn, you've crossed the finish line. But here's the thing: it's not actually a finish line. It's the start of something entirely new. And often, the very first hours of this new start take place in one of the most challenging environments imaginable for a neurodivergent person: the postnatal ward.

The transition from the delivery room or operating theater to the postnatal ward can feel abrupt. One minute, you are in a relatively controlled environment focused on a single task—birth. The next, you are wheeled into a space that often feels like sensory chaos. For someone whose brain processes information differently, this immediate postpartum period is incredibly sensitive. Your physical body is recovering, your hormones are shifting dramatically, and your sensory cup is likely already full, if not overflowing.

Many new parents describe the postnatal ward as a blurry, exhausting haze. But when you add autism or ADHD into the mix, that haze can become a thunderstorm. Understanding the specific challenges of this environment is the first step to managing it. It's not about making the ward perfect. (Let's be real, that's probably not happening.) It's about finding ways to protect your energy, advocate for your needs, and create pockets of calm amidst the storm.

**The sensory assault of the postnatal ward**

Let's talk about what a typical postnatal ward actually feels like. If you haven't been in one before, the reality can be jarring.

Hospitals are not designed for rest. That sounds counterintuitive, doesn't it? But they are designed for monitoring, efficiency, and safety. This means constant activity, 24 hours a day. For a neurodivergent person, particularly someone who is autistic, the sensory input can be overwhelming.

Think about the noise. There are the constant beeps and alarms from medical equipment. Some are urgent; many are not. But your brain, already on high alert, has trouble telling the difference. There are the sounds of other babies crying, sometimes right next to you, separated only by a thin curtain. There are staff conversations, the clatter of food trays, the squeak of shoes on linoleum floors, and the loud rumble of cleaning carts. Studies have shown that noise levels in hospitals often exceed recommendations, which significantly impacts patient recovery and stress levels (O'Shea et al., 2021). For someone with auditory sensitivity, this isn't just annoying; it can be physically painful.

Then there are the lights. Hospital lighting is typically harsh, bright, and fluorescent. It buzzes. It flickers. And often, you don't have full control over it. In a shared room, the main lights might be switched on at 6 AM for morning rounds, regardless of whether you finally managed to fall asleep 30 minutes earlier.

And the interruptions? They are endless. Vital sign checks, pain medication offers, pediatrician visits, lactation consultant rounds, hearing screenings for the baby, meal deliveries, cleaning staff, and visitors (both yours and your roommates'). It feels like every time you try to rest, feed your baby, or simply process what has happened, someone pulls back the curtain. This lack of predictability is incredibly taxing on the autistic brain, which thrives on routine and knowing what comes next. It also constantly breaks the focus of an ADHD brain trying to master a new skill like feeding.

**Shared spaces and the loss of control**

A major stressor on the postnatal ward is the lack of privacy. In many healthcare systems, private rooms are rare or expensive. Most new parents find themselves in shared rooms, often with two, three, or sometimes even more families.

Sharing a space means managing the sensory input of others. It means navigating different cultural expectations about noise and visitors. It means smelling your roommate's dinner when you are feeling nauseous. But perhaps most difficult is the feeling of being observed.

Masking—the act of hiding neurodivergent traits to fit in—takes a huge amount of energy. In the immediate postpartum period, you simply don't have that energy. Yet, the pressure to perform "good parenting" is intense. When you are in a shared space, you might feel like you have to suppress stimming (self-soothing movements), manage your reactions to sensory overload, and interact socially with strangers, all while recovering from a major medical event. It's exhausting.

Let's look at Maya's experience. Maya is autistic and gave birth to her first child via an unplanned C-section. Physically, she was in pain and restricted in her movement. Sensorily, she was completely overwhelmed. She was placed in a four-bed room.

"It was a nightmare," she shared. "The woman next to me had the TV on loud all day. The woman across from me had about ten visitors who were all talking over each other. I couldn't sleep. I couldn't even look at my baby without feeling panicked. Every time a nurse came in, I tried to seem calm, but inside I was shutting down. I started dissociating. I couldn't process anything they were telling me about medication or feeding. By the second day, I just pulled the sheet over my head and refused to talk. They thought I had severe postpartum depression, but honestly? It was the environment."

Maya's reaction is understandable. When the environment is too intense, the brain protects itself by shutting down. Recognizing this as a sensory issue, rather than a mood issue or an inability to cope, is crucial.

**The Golden Hour adapted for the sensory reality**

You've probably heard of the "Golden Hour." This refers to the first hour or so after birth, often idealized as a time for immediate skin-to-skin contact, the first feed, and quiet bonding. It's presented as essential for attachment. And yes, skin-to-skin contact has many benefits for both the parent and the baby, including regulating the baby's temperature and heart rate (Moore et al., 2016).

However. And this is a big however. The pressure to perform the Golden Hour perfectly can be immense. What if you are touch-averse? What if the sensation of a sticky, wet newborn on your skin makes you want to crawl out of your own body? What if you are so overloaded by the birth itself that any further sensory input is too much?

Here's the truth: It is okay if you don't want immediate skin-to-skin contact. It is okay if you need a moment to breathe. Your attachment with your child is not built in one hour. It is built over a lifetime.

**Challenges with skin-to-skin when touch-averse**

Touch aversion is common among neurodivergent people. It doesn't mean you don't love your baby. It means that the sensation of touch can be overwhelming or uncomfortable. In the postpartum period, this can be heightened. Your body has been through a lot. You might feel "touched out" from the constant medical interventions during labor.

If the idea of skin-to-skin makes you anxious, forcing yourself to do it because "you should" is counterproductive. If you are stressed and dysregulated, your baby will pick up on that. A calm parent is better than a stressed parent doing skin-to-skin.

So, how do we adapt the Golden Hour?

1. **Redefine contact:** Skin-to-skin doesn't have to mean full chest contact. Maybe it's holding your baby's hand. Maybe it's having the baby swaddled and placed next to you so you can look at them. Maybe it's your partner doing the skin-to-skin while you rest nearby.

2. **Use barriers:** If you want the closeness but dislike the sensation of skin, try placing a thin, soft blanket or sheet between you and the baby. You still get the proximity and the warmth.

3. **Titrate exposure:** Start small. Maybe you can manage five minutes of skin-to-skin, then take a break. That's perfectly fine. You can build up gradually as you feel comfortable.

4. **Focus on other senses:** Bonding isn't just about touch. It's about your voice, your smell, and your presence. Talk to your baby. Look at them. Let them get used to you in ways that feel manageable for your sensory system.

The key is communication. You need to tell your medical team *before* the baby is born that immediate skin-to-skin might be difficult for you. We talked about this in the birth planning chapters, but it bears repeating. Use clear language. "Due to my sensory processing needs, I may need a break before initiating skin-to-skin. Please wrap the baby and hand them to my partner first."

Don't let anyone shame you for this. This is about making the transition into parenthood sustainable for you.

**Advocating for environmental adjustments on the ward**

Once you are on the postnatal ward, the advocacy work continues. Your birth plan doesn't expire once the baby is born. It should include a section on postpartum care. When you arrive on the ward, you or your support person needs to communicate your needs to the staff.

It can feel difficult to ask for special treatment. We are often socialized, especially women and marginalized genders, to be compliant patients. To not make a fuss. But these adjustments are not luxuries. They are necessary accommodations for a neurological difference.

Here are some specific adjustments you can request:

**Private rooms**

This is the single most helpful adjustment for many neurodivergent parents. A private room gives you control over your environment. You can dim the lights, control the noise level, and manage visitors without negotiating with roommates.

If you are in a system where private rooms are available, request one as early as possible. If they cost money, consider if it is a worthwhile investment in your mental health. If they are typically reserved for specific medical needs, make the case that your neurodivergence *is* a medical need. A letter from your doctor or therapist explaining why a private room is necessary to prevent sensory overload and support your mental health can be very helpful here.

In situations where a private room is absolutely not available, you can still ask to be placed in the quietest corner of the ward, perhaps away from the nursing station or the main entrance.

**Structured interruptions**

The constant, unpredictable interruptions are a major source of stress. You can ask the staff to structure their interactions with you.

1. **Clustering care:** This means doing several tasks at once, rather than coming in repeatedly. For example, ask them to check your vitals, give you medication, and check the baby's diaper all in one visit.

2. **Predictable schedules:** Ask when rounds typically happen. Knowing when to expect interruptions can help you mentally prepare.

3. **Do not disturb:** Ask for a sign on your door or curtain during specific times when you need to rest. You can say, "I need to rest between 2 PM and 4 PM. Unless it is an emergency, please do not disturb me."

4. **Clear communication:** Ask staff to knock or announce themselves quietly before entering your space, rather than abruptly pulling back the curtain.

## Sensory environment modifications

Even in a shared room, there are small changes that can make a big difference.

1. **Lighting:** Ask if the main lights can be kept dimmed, and use a smaller task light if needed. Bring your own eye mask or a scarf to block out light.

2. **Noise:** Noise-canceling headphones are your best friend on the postnatal ward. You can wear them while resting, even while feeding your baby. Loop earplugs, which reduce the volume without blocking all sound, can also be helpful if you need to be able to hear your baby but want to minimize background noise.

3. **Smell:** Bring your own toiletries with scents that you find calming or neutral. Essential oils on a cotton ball can help mask unpleasant hospital smells.

4. **Touch:** Bring your own comfortable clothing, pillow, and blanket. The texture of hospital linens can be scratchy and uncomfortable.

Remember, you are not being difficult by asking for these things. You are proactively managing your environment so you can recover and care for your baby.

## Handovers and the continuity of care challenge

Here's a scenario that happens all the time. You spend hours explaining your needs to a lovely, understanding nurse during the day shift. They put accommodations in place. They get it. Then, 7 PM rolls around, the shift changes, and you are back to square one. The night nurse comes in, flips on the bright lights, and starts talking loudly.

Handovers—the process of transferring patient information between shifts—are notoriously tricky in busy hospital environments. Information gets lost. Nuance gets missed. And often, information about neurodiversity needs is the first thing to be dropped if it's not seen as medically critical.

Ensuring continuity of neurodiversity-affirming care across shifts is a major challenge. It requires proactive strategies on your part.

### The communication passport

One tool that can be incredibly helpful is a "communication passport" or a "patient preference sheet." This is a simple, one-page document that summarizes your neurodivergence, your communication preferences, and your specific needs. It's more immediate than a birth plan, which can be long and detailed.

Your passport should include:

- **My diagnosis/identity:** (e.g., "I am autistic," or "I have ADHD and sensory processing differences.")

- **How this affects me:** (e.g., "I am sensitive to bright lights and loud noises," "I need clear, direct communication," "I may have difficulty processing verbal instructions when overwhelmed.")

- **What helps me:** (e.g., "Please keep lights dimmed," "Please cluster care to minimize interruptions," "Please speak quietly and one person at a time," "Please allow me to wear headphones.")

- **My feeding plan:** (e.g., "I am formula feeding," or "I need support with breastfeeding, but I am touch-averse.")

Keep this passport visible. Tape it to the wall above your bed. Hand it to every new staff member who enters your space. This saves you the energy of having to explain yourself repeatedly. It also gives staff clear, actionable information on how to support you.

### The role of the support person

If you have a partner or a support person with you, their role in ensuring continuity of care is critical. They need to be the gatekeeper and the advocate. When a new staff member comes in, your support person can take the lead. "Hi, this is Alex. Just so you know, Alex is autistic and needs a quiet environment. We have a preference sheet here. Can you please make sure this is noted in the handover?"

This is especially important if you are non-speaking or have difficulty communicating when stressed. Your support person needs to be prepared to step in and firmly, but politely, reiterate your needs.

**Navigating inconsistent advice**

Another challenge related to handovers is inconsistent advice. The day nurse tells you one thing about feeding. The night nurse tells you the opposite. The pediatrician says something else entirely. This is confusing for any new parent, but for neurodivergent people, it can be incredibly distressing.

Autistic individuals often prefer clear rules and guidelines. Contradictory information can cause anxiety and make it difficult to know what to do. ADHD individuals might feel overwhelmed by the conflicting options and struggle to make a decision.

When you receive inconsistent advice, here's what you can do:

1. **Ask for the evidence:** Politely ask the staff member to explain the reasoning behind their advice. "That's interesting. The previous nurse suggested X. Can you explain why you recommend Y?"

2. **Identify your priority:** What is most important to you right now? Is it rest? Is it establishing feeding? Choose the advice that aligns best with your immediate goals and your sensory needs.

3. **Go with your gut:** You know your body and your baby best. If a piece of advice feels wrong or unsustainable for you, you don't have to take it.

4.  **Seek a tie-breaker:** If you are truly stuck, ask to speak with the charge nurse or the attending physician to get a definitive answer.

The immediate postpartum period on the ward is about survival. It's about getting through those first few days in an environment that is often not set up for your success. Be gentle with yourself. Advocate for your needs. And remember that this phase is temporary. You will go home. And once you are home, you can start creating an environment that truly supports you and your new family.

---

**Key Takeaways from the Immediate Postpartum Period**

- The postnatal ward is often a challenging sensory environment due to noise, bright lights, constant interruptions, and shared spaces.

- Sensory overload in the hospital can lead to stress, anxiety, and shutdown, impacting recovery and bonding.

- The "Golden Hour" and skin-to-skin contact should be adapted to your sensory needs. Touch aversion is valid, and attachment is not built in a single hour.

- Advocacy continues after birth. Request environmental adjustments such as private rooms, clustered care, and modifications to lighting and noise levels.

- Handovers between shifts often lead to loss of information. Use a communication passport and rely on your support person to ensure continuity of neurodiversity-affirming care.

- Navigate inconsistent advice by asking for evidence, identifying your priorities, and trusting your intuition.

# Chapter 11: Feeding Support and Neurodivergence

Once you start to settle in—whether you are still in the hospital or have transitioned home—the reality of feeding your newborn takes center stage. It's relentless. Newborns eat all the time. Every two to three hours, around the clock. And while feeding is a natural process, it rarely comes easily.

There is so much pressure surrounding how we feed our babies. "Breast is best" is a message we hear constantly. And while breastfeeding or chestfeeding has known benefits, the conversation often lacks nuance. It ignores the reality that for many people, it is incredibly difficult. And for neurodivergent parents, the challenges are often magnified.

When we talk about feeding difficulties, we usually focus on the mechanics: the latch, the supply, the baby's weight gain. But we rarely talk about the sensory experience of feeding. We don't talk about how executive function challenges impact our ability to manage the logistics of feeding. We don't talk about how neurodivergence affects our relationship with our bodies and how that impacts our feeding choices.

This chapter is about looking at feeding through a neurodivergent lens. It's about validating your experiences, offering practical strategies, and emphasizing that the most important thing is a fed baby and a healthy parent. Whether you choose to breastfeed, chestfeed, pump, formula feed, or use donor milk, your choices are valid. The goal is to find a feeding method that is sustainable for you and your family.

**The intense sensory world of breastfeeding and chestfeeding**

For many neurodivergent people, the sensory aspects of breastfeeding or chestfeeding are the biggest hurdle. It's not about the mechanics. It's about how it *feels*.

**Touch aversion and feeling "touched out"**

We talked about touch aversion in the context of the Golden Hour. But it continues to be a factor throughout the feeding journey. Breastfeeding is an incredibly intimate, physical experience. You are holding your baby close to your body, often skin-to-skin. The sensation of the baby rooting, the latch, the suckling—it can all be overwhelming.

If you have a sensory system that is easily overloaded by touch, this constant physical contact can lead to feeling "touched out." This is a state where any further physical contact feels unbearable. You might feel irritable, anxious, or even angry when the baby latches. You might want to pull away or push the baby off.

This can lead to a lot of guilt and shame. "Why can't I enjoy this?" "Doesn't this mean I don't love my baby?" Let me be very clear: Feeling touched out has nothing to do with your love for your child. It is a physiological response to sensory overload.

Let's look at Chloe's experience. Chloe has sensory processing differences and has always been sensitive to light touch. When she started breastfeeding her son, she struggled.

"The latch itself didn't hurt," she explained. "But the sensation of his mouth on my nipple made my skin crawl. It was like nails on a chalkboard, but on my body. I would grit my teeth and try to get through it, but I dreaded every feed. I felt so guilty. Everyone talks about how beautiful and bonding breastfeeding is, but for me, it felt like torture."

Chloe's experience is common. If you are struggling with touch aversion, here are some strategies that might help:

1. **Use barriers:** Nipple shields can sometimes change the sensation of the latch, making it more tolerable. Wearing clothing that minimizes skin-to-skin contact can also help.

2. **Change positions:** Experiment with different feeding positions. Some positions, like the side-lying position, might feel less restrictive and reduce the amount of full-body contact.

3. **Grounding techniques:** During feeds, try to focus on something else that grounds you. Listen to an audiobook or music. Squeeze a stress ball. Focus on deep breathing.

4. **Take breaks:** If you feel overwhelmed, it is okay to unlatch the baby, take a moment to regulate yourself, and then try again.

## Auditory sensitivity and the sounds of feeding

It's not just touch. The sounds of breastfeeding can also be triggering. The sound of the baby suckling, swallowing, smacking their lips—it can be grating for someone with auditory sensitivity or misophonia (a condition where specific sounds trigger strong emotional or physiological responses).

If you find yourself getting agitated by the sounds of feeding, try using earplugs or headphones. Playing white noise or calming music can also help mask the triggering sounds.

## The sensory experience of milk ejection

The let-down reflex, or milk ejection reflex, is the physical process of milk being released from the breasts. For some people, this feels like a tingling or warming sensation. For others, it can be painful.

But there is another aspect of milk ejection that is rarely discussed: Dysphoric Milk Ejection Reflex (D-MER). D-MER is a condition where the release of milk triggers a sudden onset of negative emotions, such as sadness, anxiety, irritability, or even dread (Ureño et al., 2019). This is a physiological response, likely related to the sudden drop in dopamine that occurs during milk ejection. It's not postpartum depression. It's a specific, temporary response to the feeding process.

D-MER can be particularly distressing for neurodivergent people who already struggle with emotional regulation. If you experience a sudden wave of negative emotions right before or during a feed, know that you are not alone and that this is a recognized phenomenon. For many people, simply knowing that it has a name and a physiological cause can help reduce the distress.

**ADHD and the logistical puzzle of feeding**

For parents with ADHD, the challenges of feeding are often less about the sensory experience and more about the logistics, routine, and focus required.

**Time blindness and the challenge of routine**

Newborns need to eat frequently. But keeping track of time can be incredibly difficult for people with ADHD. Time blindness—the inability to accurately perceive the passage of time—means that you might look up and realize that four hours have passed since the last feed, even though it felt like 30 minutes.

This can cause a lot of anxiety, especially if you are worried about your baby's weight gain. Establishing a routine can feel impossible when your brain is constantly jumping from one thing to the next.

Here are some strategies for managing time blindness and routine:

1. **Use technology:** Set alarms and reminders on your phone for every feed. Use a feeding tracking app to log when the baby eats, which side they ate on, and their diaper output. This externalizes the information so you don't have to rely on your working memory.

2. **Anchor feeds to other activities:** Instead of relying solely on the clock, try anchoring feeds to other daily activities. For

example, feed the baby when you wake up, before you eat lunch, and before you go to bed.

3. **Be flexible:** Instead of aiming for a rigid schedule, focus on a rhythm. Recognize that some days will be more structured than others, and that's okay.

## Challenges with focus and distraction

Breastfeeding requires you to sit still and focus on the task at hand for a significant amount of time. This can be very difficult for people with ADHD who have a high need for stimulation and struggle with boredom.

You might find yourself getting restless during feeds, constantly reaching for your phone, or trying to multitask. This can lead to distraction, which can impact the effectiveness of the feed. The baby might also pick up on your restlessness and become fussy.

Here's how to manage focus challenges:

1. **Create a feeding station:** Set up a comfortable spot with everything you need within reach: water, snacks, your phone, a book, the remote control. This minimizes the need to get up and interrupt the feed.

2. **Engage your senses:** If you need stimulation, try listening to an engaging podcast or watching a show during feeds. This can help keep you focused on the task while also meeting your need for input.

3. **Practice mindfulness (but ADHD style):** Traditional mindfulness meditation might be difficult, but you can practice mindful observation. Notice the details of your baby. The way their hair curls. The sound of their breathing. This can help keep you present in the moment.

## Impulsivity and feeding decisions

ADHD impulsivity can also impact feeding decisions. You might find yourself getting frustrated quickly if breastfeeding isn't working and impulsively deciding to switch to formula, only to regret the decision later. Or you might find yourself buying every feeding gadget on the market in the hope of finding a quick fix.

It's important to slow down and make intentional decisions about feeding. Talk to a lactation consultant or a trusted healthcare provider before making any major changes. Give yourself time to adjust and troubleshoot before giving up on a method if it is something you want to continue.

**Executive function support for bottle feeding**

Bottle feeding—whether with expressed milk or formula—is often presented as the easier option. But it comes with its own set of executive function challenges. It requires planning, organization, and consistent effort to manage the logistics.

**The hidden labor of sterilization and organization**

Bottle feeding involves a lot of steps. You need to sterilize the bottles and pump parts. You need to prepare the formula or thaw the expressed milk. You need to remember to bring enough supplies when you leave the house. You need to keep track of how long the milk has been sitting out.

This is a lot for a brain that struggles with executive function, especially when you are sleep-deprived and overwhelmed.

Let's break down the organizational strategies that can help:

1. **Simplify the process:** You don't need fancy bottle warmers or sterilizers. A pot of boiling water works just fine for sterilization. If you are formula feeding, pre-measure the powder into containers so you can quickly mix a bottle when needed.

2. **Create systems:** Have a designated area for all the feeding supplies. Use bins to organize bottles, nipples, pump parts, and formula.

3. **Batch tasks:** Instead of washing bottles one by one throughout the day, wash them all at once at the end of the day. Prepare a batch of formula for the day and store it in the refrigerator.

4. **The "good enough" approach:** It is okay if the bottles are not perfectly organized. It is okay if you forget to sterilize a pump part once in a while. Aim for "good enough" rather than perfection.

## Pumping and the executive function load

Exclusive pumping adds another layer of complexity. You are essentially doing double duty: feeding the baby with a bottle and pumping to maintain your milk supply. This requires a significant amount of time, organization, and mental energy.

Pumping requires assembling the pump parts, sitting down to pump for 15-30 minutes every few hours, storing the milk, and then washing the parts. It's a relentless cycle.

If you are exclusively pumping, here are some tips to manage the executive function load:

1. **Invest in efficiency:** A hands-free pumping bra allows you to do other things while pumping. Having multiple sets of pump parts means you don't have to wash them after every session.

2. **Automate the schedule:** Use alarms and reminders to keep you on track with your pumping schedule.

3. **Be realistic about the commitment:** Exclusive pumping is hard. If it becomes too overwhelming, it is okay to supplement with formula or switch to formula entirely.

## Recognizing and addressing feeding aversion or dysphoria

Sometimes, the challenges with feeding go beyond sensory overload or executive function difficulties. For some neurodivergent people, the act of feeding itself can trigger intense negative emotions or even gender dysphoria.

## Feeding aversion

Feeding aversion is a phenomenon where the parent experiences intense negative emotions, such as anger, agitation, or disgust, when the baby latches (Yate, 2017). It is often associated with feeling overwhelmed, touched out, or trapped.

Feeding aversion can be incredibly distressing. It can lead to feelings of guilt, shame, and isolation. If you are experiencing feeding aversion, it is important to seek support. A lactation consultant or a therapist who understands neurodivergence can help you identify the triggers and develop coping strategies.

Sometimes, the only solution is to reduce the frequency of feeds or stop breastfeeding entirely. And that is okay. Your mental health matters more than how you feed your baby.

## Gender dysphoria and feeding

For transgender and non-binary parents, chestfeeding can be a complex experience. For some, it can be a gender-affirming experience. For others, it can trigger intense gender dysphoria related to their chest.

If you are experiencing gender dysphoria related to feeding, it is essential to prioritize your mental health. You might choose to bind your chest and formula feed. You might choose to pump and bottle feed to minimize the physical contact with your chest. You might choose to use a supplemental nursing system (SNS) to provide milk at the chest without relying on your own supply.

There is no right way to feed your baby. The best method is the one that supports your mental health and allows you to bond with your child in a way that feels authentic to you.

## Finding neurodiversity-affirming feeding support

The challenge is that much of the standard feeding support is not neurodiversity-affirming. Lactation consultants might not understand sensory processing differences or executive function challenges.

They might push breastfeeding at all costs, ignoring the impact on your mental health.

When seeking feeding support, look for providers who:

- Understand and validate your sensory experiences.
- Offer practical strategies for managing executive function challenges.
- Respect your autonomy and your feeding choices.
- Prioritize your mental health alongside your feeding goals.

Don't be afraid to ask questions and advocate for your needs. If a provider is not supportive or understanding, find another one. You deserve compassionate, individualized care.

**The bottom line on feeding**

Feeding a newborn is hard work. When you add neurodivergence into the mix, it can feel overwhelming. Whether you are struggling with sensory overload, executive function challenges, feeding aversion, or dysphoria, your experiences are valid.

Be compassionate with yourself. Let go of the pressure to perform feeding perfectly. Focus on finding a sustainable solution that works for you and your family. A fed baby and a healthy parent—that is the only goal that truly matters.

---

**Key Takeaways on Feeding Support**

- The sensory aspects of breastfeeding/chestfeeding, such as touch aversion, auditory sensitivity, and D-MER, can be significant challenges for neurodivergent parents.
- ADHD impacts feeding through challenges with routine, time management (time blindness), focus, and impulsivity. Externalizing information through technology and systems is key.

- Bottle feeding and pumping require significant executive function skills. Simplifying processes, creating systems, and batching tasks can help manage the load.

- Feeding aversion and gender dysphoria are real and distressing experiences. Prioritizing your mental health is essential, even if it means changing your feeding method.

- Seek out neurodiversity-affirming feeding support that respects your autonomy, validates your experiences, and offers practical, individualized strategies.

# Chapter 12: Perinatal Mental Health and Neurodivergent Burnout

We've talked about the physical recovery, the sensory environment of the hospital, and the challenges of feeding. Now, we need to talk about what's happening inside your mind. The perinatal period—the time during pregnancy and the first year after birth—is a time of immense vulnerability for mental health. And for neurodivergent people, the risks are even higher.

It's easy to see why. The transition to parenthood is a massive life change. It involves sleep deprivation, hormonal fluctuations, identity shifts, and a steep learning curve. Add to that the sensory overload, the executive function demands, and the pressure to mask and conform to neurotypical expectations of parenting, and it's a perfect storm for mental health challenges.

But here's the tricky part: mental health issues in neurodivergent people often look different than in neurotypical people. Standard screening tools might miss the signs. Healthcare providers might misinterpret your symptoms. And you might struggle to articulate what you are experiencing.

This chapter is about understanding the unique mental health landscape of the perinatal period for neurodivergent parents. It's about recognizing the signs of Perinatal Mood and Anxiety Disorders (PMADs), distinguishing them from neurodivergent burnout, and finding the right support. Because you don't have to go through this alone.

**The heightened risk of PMADs for neurodivergent parents**

Let's start with the facts. Neurodivergent people are more likely to experience mental health challenges throughout their lives. And the perinatal period is no exception.

Research shows that autistic individuals have significantly higher rates of perinatal depression and anxiety compared to the general population (Pohl et al., 2020). Similarly, individuals with ADHD are at increased risk for postpartum depression and anxiety (Andersson et al., 2023).

Why is the risk higher? There are several factors at play.

1. **Sensory overload:** The constant sensory input of caring for a newborn—the crying, the touch, the smells—can quickly lead to sensory overload, which is directly linked to anxiety and stress.

2. **Executive function demands:** The organizational and planning skills required for parenting can be overwhelming for people with executive function challenges, leading to feelings of inadequacy and failure.

3. **Masking and social pressure:** The pressure to perform parenting "correctly" and conform to social expectations can lead to increased masking, which is mentally exhausting and contributes to burnout and depression.

4. **Communication challenges:** Difficulty communicating needs and experiences to healthcare providers and support systems can lead to isolation and lack of adequate support.

5. **Hormonal sensitivity:** Neurodivergent people may be more sensitive to the hormonal fluctuations of the perinatal period, which can impact mood and emotional regulation.

**Recognizing the signs of PMADs**

PMADs encompass a range of conditions, including perinatal depression, anxiety, obsessive-compulsive disorder (OCD), and post-traumatic stress disorder (PTSD).

The signs of PMADs can be subtle and easily dismissed as "normal" new parent stress. But if you are experiencing any of the following symptoms for more than two weeks, it's important to seek help:

- Persistent sadness, hopelessness, or emptiness.

- Severe anxiety, panic attacks, or constant worry.

- Intrusive thoughts or images that are distressing (this is common in perinatal OCD).

- Irritability, anger, or rage.

- Difficulty bonding with your baby.

- Loss of interest in activities you usually enjoy.

- Changes in sleep or appetite (beyond the usual newborn sleep deprivation).

- Feelings of worthlessness or excessive guilt.

- Thoughts of self-harm or suicide.

If you are having thoughts of self-harm or suicide, seek immediate help. Contact a crisis hotline or go to the nearest emergency room.

**The unique presentation of PMADs in neurodivergent people**

Here's where it gets complicated. In neurodivergent people, PMADs might not fit the typical mold.

For example, in autistic individuals, depression might not present as sadness, but rather as increased irritability, withdrawal, or a loss of skills. Anxiety might manifest as increased sensory sensitivity, more rigid adherence to routines, or increased stimming.

In individuals with ADHD, depression might look like extreme executive dysfunction, inability to initiate tasks, or emotional dysregulation. Anxiety might present as restlessness, racing thoughts, or hyperfocus on specific worries.

This is why standard screening tools, which are designed for neurotypical presentations, often miss the signs of PMADs in neurodivergent people. It's essential to trust your own experience. If you feel like something is wrong, even if you can't articulate it perfectly, seek help.

**The crucial distinction: Postnatal Depression vs. Neurodivergent Burnout**

This is perhaps one of the most important distinctions to understand. Many neurodivergent parents are misdiagnosed with postpartum depression when what they are actually experiencing is autistic burnout or ADHD paralysis.

**Autistic Burnout**

Autistic burnout is a state of intense physical, mental, and emotional exhaustion that results from the chronic stress of masking and navigating a world designed for neurotypical people (Raymaker et al., 2020). It is characterized by:

- **Loss of skills:** Difficulty with tasks that were previously manageable, such as communication, executive function, or self-care.

- **Increased sensory sensitivity:** Even minor sensory input can feel overwhelming.

- **Reduced tolerance for social interaction:** Increased need for solitude and withdrawal.

- **Increased autistic traits:** More noticeable stimming, difficulty with eye contact, or more rigid thinking.

- **Physical exhaustion:** Deep fatigue that is not relieved by sleep.

In the postpartum period, the demands of parenting, the sensory overload, and the pressure to mask can quickly lead to autistic burnout.

Let's look at Jessica's story. Jessica was diagnosed with autism as an adult. When she had her baby, she found herself struggling. She was exhausted, overwhelmed, and unable to keep up with the household tasks. She stopped talking as much and found herself getting easily agitated by her baby's crying.

Her doctor screened her for postpartum depression and prescribed antidepressants. But they didn't help. In fact, they made her feel numb and disconnected. It wasn't until she connected with an autistic therapist that she realized she was experiencing autistic burnout.

"It wasn't that I was sad," she explained. "It was that my brain had shut down. I had nothing left to give. I needed sensory breaks, practical support, and permission to stop masking. I didn't need medication. I needed accommodation."

## ADHD Paralysis

ADHD paralysis, also known as executive dysfunction overwhelm, is a state where the brain is so overwhelmed by the demands of tasks that it shuts down, making it impossible to initiate or complete tasks. It is characterized by:

- **Inability to prioritize:** Everything feels equally important, leading to decision fatigue.

- **Mental freezing:** Feeling stuck and unable to move forward, even on simple tasks.

- **Procrastination:** Avoiding tasks because they feel too overwhelming.

- **Emotional dysregulation:** Increased irritability, anxiety, or frustration.

In the postpartum period, the sheer volume of tasks involved in caring for a newborn can trigger ADHD paralysis. You know what you need to do—feed the baby, change the diaper, wash the bottles—but you can't seem to make yourself do it.

## Why the distinction matters

Distinguishing between depression and burnout/paralysis is critical because the treatment approaches are different.

If you have postpartum depression, the treatment might involve therapy, medication, and social support.

If you are experiencing autistic burnout or ADHD paralysis, the focus is on reducing the demands, managing sensory input, and implementing strategies to support executive function. Antidepressants might not be helpful and could even exacerbate the symptoms.

How do you tell the difference? It's not always easy, as there can be overlap. But here are some questions to ask yourself:

- **What is the primary feeling?** Is it sadness and hopelessness (depression) or exhaustion and overwhelm (burnout/paralysis)?

- **What helps?** Does social interaction make you feel better (depression) or worse (burnout)? Does rest alleviate the fatigue (depression) or not (burnout)?

- **What are the triggers?** Are the symptoms triggered by specific situations, such as sensory overload or excessive demands (burnout/paralysis), or are they pervasive (depression)?

If you suspect you are experiencing burnout or paralysis, it is essential to communicate this to your healthcare provider. Use clear language. "I think I am experiencing autistic burnout due to the sensory overload and the demands of parenting."

## The devastating impact of sensory overload and masking on mental health

We cannot talk about perinatal mental health in neurodivergent people without talking about the impact of sensory overload and masking.

## The energy cost of masking

Masking is the act of hiding your neurodivergent traits to fit into neurotypical expectations. It might involve forcing eye contact, suppressing stimming, mimicking social behaviors, or minimizing sensory discomfort.

Masking takes a huge amount of cognitive energy. It's like running a complex computer program in the background of your brain all the time. In the postpartum period, when you are already sleep-deprived and overwhelmed, the energy cost of masking is simply too high.

The pressure to mask as a parent is intense. You might feel like you have to perform "perfect parenting" in front of healthcare providers, family members, and even other parents. You might worry that if you show signs of struggle, you will be judged or deemed unfit.

This constant masking contributes significantly to burnout, anxiety, and depression. It disconnects you from your authentic self and prevents you from accessing the support you need.

## The sensory environment of early parenting

The sensory environment of early parenting is intense. The crying, the constant touch, the lack of sleep, the smells—it's a lot. For a neurodivergent person with sensory sensitivities, this environment can be incredibly dysregulating.

When your sensory system is constantly overloaded, your nervous system goes into fight-or-flight mode. This leads to increased anxiety, irritability, and stress. It makes it difficult to bond with your baby, regulate your emotions, and manage the demands of parenting.

## Creating a sensory-safe environment

Protecting your mental health means creating a sensory-safe environment for yourself. This involves:

1. **Minimizing sensory input:** Use noise-canceling headphones or earplugs. Dim the lights. Wear comfortable clothing. Create a calm, clutter-free space in your home.

2. **Taking sensory breaks:** Take regular breaks from the demands of parenting. Go for a walk alone. Take a bath. Sit in a quiet room. Even five minutes of sensory respite can make a difference.

3. **Stimming as self-regulation:** Engage in stimming behaviors that help you regulate your nervous system. Rocking, swaying, humming, using fidget toys—whatever works for you.

4. **Communicating your needs:** Tell your partner, family, and friends what you need to manage your sensory environment. Ask for help with tasks that are sensorily overwhelming.

## Tailored mental health support and referral pathways

If you are struggling with your mental health, it is essential to seek support. But not all support is created equal. Standard mental health services are often not equipped to meet the unique needs of neurodivergent people.

## What neurodiversity-affirming mental health support looks like

Neurodiversity-affirming mental health support recognizes that neurodivergence is a natural variation of human neurology, not a disorder that needs to be cured. It focuses on understanding your unique experiences, strengths, and challenges, and developing strategies that work for your brain.

A neurodiversity-affirming therapist will:

- Understand the nuances of autism and ADHD in adults.

- Validate your sensory experiences and executive function challenges.

- Recognize the impact of masking and burnout.

- Help you develop strategies for self-regulation and self-advocacy.

- Adapt their communication style to meet your needs.

**Finding the right provider**

Finding a neurodiversity-affirming provider can be challenging, but it is worth the effort. Here are some tips:

1. **Look for specialists:** Search for therapists who specialize in adult autism, ADHD, or neurodiversity.

2. **Ask about their approach:** When contacting a therapist, ask about their experience working with neurodivergent clients and their approach to therapy.

3. **Seek recommendations:** Ask for recommendations from other neurodivergent parents or online communities.

4. **Trust your gut:** If a therapist dismisses your experiences or makes you feel uncomfortable, they are not the right fit for you.

**Practical support matters too**

Mental health support isn't just about therapy. It's also about practical support. Reducing the demands on you is essential for recovery from burnout and PMADs.

This might involve:

- **Hiring help:** If you can afford it, hire a postpartum doula, a cleaner, or a babysitter.

- **Asking for help:** Ask your partner, family, and friends for specific help with tasks such as cooking, cleaning, or childcare.

- **Simplifying your life:** Let go of non-essential commitments and expectations. Focus on the basics: feeding the baby, caring for yourself, and resting.

## A final word on your well-being

The transition to parenthood is a profound and challenging experience. When you are neurodivergent, the challenges are magnified. But so are the strengths. Your unique way of seeing the world, your ability to hyperfocus, your creativity, your empathy—these are all assets in your parenting journey.

If you are struggling, please know that you are not alone. You are not failing. You are navigating a complex transition with a brain that works differently. Be compassionate with yourself. Advocate for your needs. And seek the support you deserve. Your mental health matters. You matter.

---

## Key Takeaways on Perinatal Mental Health

- Neurodivergent individuals are at heightened risk for Perinatal Mood and Anxiety Disorders (PMADs) due to sensory overload, executive function demands, masking, and communication challenges.

- PMADs can present differently in neurodivergent people, making them harder to recognize with standard screening tools.

- It is crucial to distinguish between Postnatal Depression and Autistic Burnout or ADHD paralysis, as the treatment approaches are different. Burnout requires reducing demands and managing sensory input, not just medication.

- Masking and sensory overload significantly impact mental health. Creating a sensory-safe environment and reducing the pressure to mask are essential for well-being.

- Tailored mental health support is essential. Seek out neurodiversity-affirming providers who understand your unique needs and experiences. Practical support in reducing demands is also critical.

# Chapter 13: Implementing Systemic Change

We have talked a lot about individual interactions. The one-on-one care. The specific adjustments you make in the moment. And that is where the magic happens, truly. But here is the thing: relying solely on individual midwives to champion this cause is not sustainable. It is not fair either. If inclusive care depends entirely on whether Sarah or David is on shift, the system is broken.

We need change that sticks. Change that exists even when you are on vacation or having a tough day. We need systemic change.

This is about moving beyond good intentions and baking inclusivity right into the foundation of maternity services. It sounds huge, I know. Like trying to turn a massive ship with a tiny rudder. But it is possible. It happens piece by piece, policy by policy, room by room. It is about creating an environment where the right thing to do is also the easiest thing to do. We want to make neuro-affirming care the default setting, not an optional upgrade.

## Developing departmental guidelines and pathways for neurodivergent care

Policies and guidelines are the backbone of any healthcare system. They provide consistency. They ensure everyone knows what is expected. Right now, many maternity units have detailed pathways for conditions like gestational diabetes or preeclampsia. But when it comes to neurodiversity? Crickets.

This absence leaves a vacuum. And that vacuum gets filled with assumptions, biases, and inconsistent care. A neurodivergent person might have a fantastic experience on Tuesday and a traumatic one on Thursday, simply because the staff changed. We must fix this.

Creating specific pathways is not about labeling people or putting them in boxes. It is about recognizing that a standard approach does not work for everyone. A pathway is a map. It helps the care team know what adjustments might be needed, what questions to ask, and what resources to offer.

So, what does a good pathway look like?

First, it needs clear identification processes. This does not mean diagnosing people at the booking appointment. It means creating space for people to disclose their neurodivergence safely. This can be done through intake forms that explicitly ask about sensory needs, communication preferences, and any diagnosed conditions like Autism or ADHD. The language matters here. Instead of asking, "Do you have any disabilities?" try asking, "Are there any ways we can adjust the environment or our communication to make you more comfortable?"

Second, the pathway must outline standard adjustments. These are the low-hanging fruit. Things that should be offered proactively, not just when requested.

Examples of standard adjustments in a pathway:

1. **Priority booking for first or last appointments** to reduce waiting room stress.

2. **Offering a quiet waiting area** separate from the main, noisy space.

3. **Providing written information** before and after appointments to aid processing.

4. **Guaranteeing continuity of carer** whenever possible. This is huge for building trust.

5. **Sensory assessment** of the clinical environment.

Third, the pathway needs flexibility. This is the key difference between a neuro-affirming pathway and a rigid protocol. The guidelines should empower midwives to make individualized decisions based on the person in front of them. It is not a checklist; it is a toolkit.

Let's look at an example.

**Case Example: Implementing the "Purple Folder" System**

A mid-sized urban hospital noticed a rise in complaints from Autistic patients regarding inconsistent care during labor. The maternity lead, Fiona, decided to develop a specific pathway. They started by consulting with local neurodivergent advocacy groups. This is essential. Do not create policies *about* people without including those people.

Fiona's team developed the "Purple Folder" system. If a patient disclosed neurodivergence, their notes were placed in a purple folder. This was a visual cue for all staff that the neurodiversity pathway should be used.

Inside the folder was a one-page "Passport." It summarized the patient's specific needs, communication style, triggers, and calming strategies. It was written by the patient, with help from their midwife, early in pregnancy.

When a person with a purple folder arrived in the delivery suite, the pathway kicked in automatically:

- They were immediately moved to a pre-assigned quiet room with adjustable lighting.

- The midwife reviewed the Passport before entering the room.

- All communication was clear, literal, and concise.

- Non-essential staff were kept out of the room.

The impact? Complaints dropped significantly. Staff felt more confident because they had clear guidance. And patients felt heard. One Autistic mother shared, "The purple folder meant I didn't have to explain myself over and over again. They just knew."

That is the power of a clear pathway.

## The challenge of "buy-in"

Now, let's be real. Implementing new guidelines is not always smooth sailing. You will face resistance. People are busy. They are stressed. They might see this as "extra work."

How do you get buy-in?

You have to show them the "why." Explain that these pathways actually *save* time in the long run. They reduce complaints. They improve outcomes. They decrease the risk of traumatic births. When care is streamlined and tailored, appointments are more efficient, and crises are less likely (far et al., 2022).

Also, start small. Do not try to overhaul the entire system overnight. Pilot a new intake form. Trial a quiet waiting area. Gather feedback. Show the results. Success breeds success.

## Training and education for midwifery and obstetric staff

Guidelines are just pieces of paper if the staff are not trained to use them. Training is the engine that drives systemic change. And let's be clear: a one-off, hour-long lecture on Autism is not going to cut it.

We need comprehensive, ongoing education that challenges biases, deepens understanding, and builds practical skills.

What should this training cover?

It needs to go beyond the stereotypes. Autism is not just about rocking and hand-flapping. ADHD is not just about being hyperactive. Training should cover the diversity of neurodivergent experiences. It should highlight the internal experiences, like sensory overload, executive dysfunction, and emotional dysregulation.

## The content must be neuro-affirming

This is a big one. A lot of traditional medical training focuses on the deficits of neurodivergence. It uses pathologizing language. It treats neurodivergence as a problem to be solved.

Neuro-affirming training flips the script. It recognizes neurodivergence as a natural variation of the human brain. It focuses on strengths and differences, not just difficulties. It emphasizes adaptation and acceptance, not "curing" or masking (Dudley et al., 2023).

Who should deliver the training?

Neurodivergent people themselves. This is non-negotiable. Hearing directly from Autistic adults, ADHDers, and other neurodivergent individuals is the most powerful way to build empathy and understanding. They can share their lived experiences, explain what works and what does not, and answer questions authentically.

Pay them for their time and expertise. Do not expect free emotional labor.

**Practical skills development**

Training should not just be theoretical. It needs to equip staff with practical skills they can use immediately.

Key skills include:

- **Communication adjustments:** How to speak clearly, literally, and patiently. How to use visual aids. How to recognize and respect different communication styles.

- **Sensory accommodations:** How to identify sensory triggers in the environment. How to create a low-stimulus space.

- **Recognizing distress:** How to spot the signs of overload or meltdown, which might look different in neurodivergent people.

- **De-escalation strategies:** How to respond calmly and effectively when someone is distressed.

Role-playing and simulation are great tools here. They allow staff to practice these skills in a safe environment.

**Addressing implicit bias**

We all have biases. It is part of being human. But in healthcare, biases can be dangerous. Training must address implicit bias head-on.

Staff need space to reflect on their own assumptions about neurodivergence. They need to understand how these assumptions might affect their interactions with patients. This is not about shaming people. It is about bringing awareness to the unconscious patterns that drive our behavior.

## The ripple effect of training

Good training does more than just improve patient care. It also improves staff morale. When midwives and obstetricians feel equipped to handle complex situations, they feel more confident and less stressed.

I remember a seasoned obstetrician, Dr. Evans, who was initially skeptical about the need for neurodiversity training. He thought his 30 years of experience were enough. After attending a workshop led by an Autistic advocate, he told me, "I realized how much I didn't know. I've been misinterpreting distress as defiance for years."

That realization changed his practice. He became a champion for neuro-inclusive care.

Training is an investment. It costs money and time. But the return on investment is huge. It is measured in safer births, healthier families, and a more compassionate healthcare system.

## Creating "Sensory Toolkits" for birth rooms

We have talked extensively about the sensory environment of birth. The bright lights, the loud noises, the unfamiliar smells. It is overwhelming for anyone, but for a neurodivergent person, it can be unbearable.

Systemic change means making sensory accommodations readily available. We cannot rely on patients to bring their own comfort items, although many will. We need to provide resources within the birth environment itself.

Enter the "Sensory Toolkit."

A Sensory Toolkit is a box or cart filled with items designed to help manage sensory input and promote calm. It is a simple, low-cost intervention that can make a massive difference.

What goes into a Sensory Toolkit?

Think about the different sensory systems.

**Visual input:**

- **Eye masks or sunglasses:** To block out harsh fluorescent lighting.

- **Dimmer switches or lamps:** To adjust the lighting level. (If you cannot install dimmers, bring in some floor lamps with warm bulbs.)

- **Visual stim toys:** Things like lava lamps, bubble tubes, or sequin boards can be calming to look at.

**Auditory input:**

- **Noise-canceling headphones or ear defenders:** To block out background noise.

- **Earplugs:** A simpler option for reducing noise levels.

- **White noise machine:** To create a consistent, soothing sound environment.

- **Bluetooth speaker:** So patients can play their own calming music or affirmations.

**Tactile input:**

- **Weighted blankets or lap pads:** Deep pressure can be very regulating for the nervous system.

- **Fidget toys:** Things like stress balls, tangle toys, or silicone poppers can help channel restless energy.

- **Different textured fabrics:** Soft blankets, cool sheets, or textured towels.

- **Massage tools:** Simple tools for self-massage or partner massage.

## Olfactory (smell) input:

- **Essential oil diffuser with mild scents:** Lavender or chamomile can be calming. (Be careful with strong smells, as some people are sensitive to them.)

- **Scent-free wipes and cleaning products:** To minimize chemical smells.

## The implementation matters

Having the toolkit is the first step. Making sure it gets used is the second.

The toolkit should be easily accessible. It should not be locked away in a cupboard somewhere. Ideally, there should be one on every delivery suite.

Staff need to know what is in the toolkit and how to use it. Training should cover the basics of sensory processing and the purpose of each item.

And most importantly, patients need to know the toolkit is available. It should be offered proactively, not just when someone is visibly distressed. The midwife can say, "We have a box of things that might help you feel more comfortable. Would you like to take a look?"

## Case Example: The "Calm Cart" Pilot

A busy maternity unit in London decided to pilot a "Calm Cart." It was a rolling cart stocked with sensory items. They trained the midwives on how to introduce the cart to patients.

One midwife, Aisha, used the Calm Cart with an ADHD patient named Chloe. Chloe was anxious and restless during early labor. She kept getting up and pacing the room.

Aisha wheeled in the Calm Cart. Chloe immediately grabbed a weighted lap pad and a tangle toy. The deep pressure and the repetitive movement helped her settle. She was able to sit down and focus on her breathing.

Aisha said, "It was amazing to see the difference. The Calm Cart gave her something tangible to focus on. It changed the energy in the room."

The pilot was so successful that the hospital decided to implement Calm Carts in all birth rooms.

This is a perfect example of a small change with a big impact. It does not require expensive equipment or extensive training. It just requires a little thoughtfulness and creativity.

## Champion roles: Identifying Neurodiversity Leads within maternity services

Systems need leaders. They need people who are passionate about a cause and willing to drive change forward. That is where Neurodiversity Leads come in.

A Neurodiversity Lead is a designated person within the maternity service who takes responsibility for championing neuro-inclusive care. They are the go-to person for advice, support, and guidance on all things neurodiversity.

What does a Neurodiversity Lead do?

Their role is multifaceted. It involves education, advocacy, policy development, and support.

### Education and training

The Lead is responsible for organizing and delivering ongoing training for staff. They keep up-to-date with the latest research and best practices. They bring in external speakers and experts.

### Policy development and review

The Lead plays a key role in developing and reviewing departmental guidelines and pathways. They ensure that policies are neuro-affirming and reflect the needs of the local community.

## Support and consultation

The Lead is available to consult with staff on complex cases. They can provide advice on communication strategies, sensory accommodations, and individualized care planning. They also provide support to neurodivergent staff members (more on that in the next chapter).

## Advocacy and liaison

The Lead acts as a bridge between the maternity service and the local neurodivergent community. They build relationships with advocacy groups, gather feedback from patients, and ensure that the neurodivergent voice is heard at all levels of decision-making.

## Quality improvement

The Lead monitors the quality of care provided to neurodivergent patients. They conduct audits, analyze data, and identify areas for improvement.

Who makes a good Neurodiversity Lead?

Ideally, it should be someone with lived experience of neurodivergence. An Autistic midwife or an ADHD obstetrician brings a depth of understanding that cannot be learned from a textbook.

However, lived experience is not the only requirement. The Lead also needs strong leadership skills, excellent communication abilities, and a passion for inclusive care. They need to be resilient, because championing change is hard work.

## The structure of the role

This should not be an add-on to an already busy job. It needs dedicated time and resources. The Lead should have protected time to focus on their responsibilities. They should also have a budget for training, resources, and community engagement.

The role can be structured in different ways. It could be a full-time position, a part-time role, or a shared responsibility among a small team. The important thing is that the commitment is formalized and supported by management.

**The impact of a dedicated lead**

Having a dedicated Neurodiversity Lead sends a powerful message. It tells staff and patients that this issue matters. It shows that the organization is committed to providing inclusive care.

Research shows that having dedicated champion roles can significantly improve the implementation of evidence-based practices (Ploeg et al., 2007).

Let's look at an example.

**Case Example: The Impact of a Neurodiversity Midwife**

A large regional hospital appointed Maria, an Autistic midwife, as their Neurodiversity Lead. Maria was given two days a week dedicated to this role.

In her first year, Maria organized a series of workshops led by neurodivergent advocates. She developed a new pathway for Autistic patients, including a "Sensory Passport." She set up a monthly peer support group for neurodivergent parents.

The impact was profound. Staff reported feeling more confident in caring for neurodivergent patients. Patient satisfaction scores increased. And Maria felt empowered to make a real difference.

Maria shared, "Having this role means I can focus on systemic change. I'm not just firefighting anymore. I'm building something lasting."

**Moving forward with intention**

Implementing systemic change is a marathon, not a sprint. It requires sustained effort, collaboration, and commitment. But the rewards are immense.

By developing clear guidelines, providing comprehensive training, creating sensory-friendly environments, and appointing dedicated Neurodiversity Leads, we can build maternity services that are truly inclusive.

We can create a system where every neurodivergent person feels safe, respected, and supported throughout their perinatal journey.

It is not just about improving outcomes. It is about upholding basic human rights. The right to accessible healthcare. The right to bodily autonomy. The right to a dignified birth experience.

Now, let's turn our attention inward. Let's talk about the neurodivergent professionals working within these systems.

---

### Key Takeaways

- Relying on individual effort is not enough; systemic change is essential for sustainable, inclusive care.

- Departmental guidelines and pathways provide consistency and ensure neuro-affirming care is the default.

- Pathways should include safe identification processes, standard adjustments, and flexibility for individualized care.

- Training must be ongoing, neuro-affirming, and ideally led by neurodivergent individuals.

- Training should focus on practical skills, including communication adjustments, sensory accommodations, and recognizing distress.

- Sensory Toolkits are a low-cost, high-impact intervention for managing sensory input and promoting calm.

- Neurodiversity Leads are essential for driving change, providing education, developing policies, and advocating for the neurodivergent community.

- Champion roles need dedicated time, resources, and support from management.

# Chapter 14: The Neurodivergent Midwife

So far, we have focused primarily on the people receiving care. The Autistic parent navigating pregnancy. The ADHDer managing labor. But what about the people providing the care? What about the midwives, the obstetricians, the nurses, and the support staff who are themselves neurodivergent?

It is a conversation we do not have often enough. The healthcare profession, midwifery included, is built on an assumption of neurotypicality. The expectations, the environment, the workload— they are all designed for brains that function in a very specific way.

But the truth is, neurodivergent people are everywhere. Including in midwifery. And they bring unique strengths, perspectives, and challenges to the profession.

Acknowledging and supporting neurodivergent midwives is not just a matter of workplace inclusion. It is essential for the well-being of the profession and the quality of care we provide. When neurodivergent midwives thrive, the whole system benefits.

This discussion is about recognizing the reality of neurodiversity within our ranks, celebrating the strengths it brings, and addressing the very real challenges it presents. It is about creating a profession where everyone, regardless of their neurotype, can flourish.

## Acknowledging neurodiversity within the profession

The first step is simply acknowledging that we exist. For too long, neurodiversity has been a hidden reality within healthcare. People have masked their differences, fearing stigma, discrimination, and fitness-to-practice concerns.

We need to create a culture where midwives feel safe to disclose their neurodivergence. This starts with open and honest conversations. It starts with leadership acknowledging the presence of neurodivergent staff and valuing their contributions.

Why are neurodivergent people drawn to midwifery?

It might seem counterintuitive. Midwifery is a high-stress, sensory-intense profession. It requires constant communication, rapid decision-making, and emotional regulation.

But look closer. Midwifery also aligns with many neurodivergent strengths.

Many Autistic people have a strong sense of social justice and a desire to advocate for others. They often have an intense focus and attention to detail, which is crucial in clinical practice. They can also be highly empathetic, contrary to the stereotypes, feeling the emotions of others deeply.

ADHDers often thrive in dynamic environments where no two days are the same. They are often creative problem-solvers, able to think on their feet and adapt quickly to changing situations. Their ability to hyperfocus can be a superpower during emergencies.

Dyslexic midwives may have strong visual-spatial skills and pattern recognition abilities. They often excel at hands-on skills and holistic care.

When we recognize these strengths, we start to see neurodiversity not as a liability, but as an asset to the profession.

### The prevalence of neurodivergence in healthcare

We do not have exact statistics on the prevalence of neurodivergence among midwives. But we know that around 15-20% of the general population is neurodivergent (Doyle, 2020). There is no reason to believe the prevalence is lower in midwifery. In fact, it might even be higher, given the vocational nature of the profession.

Research into neurodiversity among nurses suggests that a significant minority identify as neurodivergent. A UK study found that 7.4% of nurses reported having a diagnosis of dyslexia, dyspraxia, Autism, or ADHD (Corden et al., 2021). And this likely underestimates the true prevalence, given the barriers to diagnosis and disclosure.

We need more research specifically focused on midwifery. But the anecdotal evidence is overwhelming. Neurodivergent midwives are here. They are doing the work. And they need to be seen.

### Creating a culture of disclosure

How do we create an environment where midwives feel safe to disclose?

1. **Visible allies and role models:** Seeing senior midwives who are openly neurodivergent makes a huge difference. It shows that neurodivergence is not a barrier to career progression.

2. **Inclusive policies:** Workplace policies should explicitly mention neurodiversity and outline the process for requesting accommodations.

3. **Positive language:** Using neuro-affirming language when discussing neurodiversity helps reduce stigma.

4. **Training for managers:** Managers need to be trained on how to support neurodivergent staff and respond appropriately to disclosures.

It is not just about formal disclosure to HR. It is also about creating a culture where colleagues can share their experiences and support each other informally.

### Strengths and challenges of being an Autistic or ADHD midwife

Being a neurodivergent midwife is a double-edged sword. It comes with unique strengths that can enhance practice. But it also comes with significant challenges that can lead to burnout and distress.

Let's break it down.

**The Autistic midwife**

**Strengths:**

- **Attention to detail:** Autistic midwives often notice small details that others might miss. They can be meticulous with documentation and clinical procedures.

- **Deep focus (Hyperfocus):** When engaged in a task, Autistic midwives can maintain intense focus for long periods. This is invaluable during complex births or research projects.

- **Pattern recognition:** Autistic brains are often wired to spot patterns. This can help in identifying clinical trends or anticipating complications.

- **Honesty and integrity:** Autistic people often have a strong moral compass and a commitment to honesty. They can be fierce advocates for their patients.

- **Empathy:** Many Autistic midwives experience hyper-empathy, feeling the emotions of others intensely. This can foster deep connections with patients.

**Challenges:**

- **Sensory overload:** The birth environment is a sensory nightmare. The bright lights, the loud noises, the strong smells, the constant interruptions. This can lead to exhaustion, anxiety, and meltdowns.

- **Communication differences:** Autistic midwives may struggle with the nuanced, indirect communication styles common in healthcare. They may be perceived as blunt or rude, even when they do not mean to be.

- **Social interactions:** Navigating the complex social dynamics of a busy maternity unit can be exhausting. Small talk, office politics, and networking can be draining.

- **Executive dysfunction:** Difficulty with planning, prioritizing, and time management can be a major challenge in a fast-paced environment.

- **Emotional regulation:** The intensity of the work, combined with hyper-empathy, can lead to emotional exhaustion and vicarious trauma.

## Case Example: Sarah, the Autistic Midwife

Sarah is a newly qualified midwife. She is passionate about evidence-based practice and excels at clinical skills. She can spot the early signs of fetal distress long before the monitors pick it up.

But she struggles with the social aspects of the job. During handovers, she often interrupts her colleagues to correct inaccuracies. She does not mean to be rude; she just values precision. Her colleagues perceive her as arrogant and difficult to work with.

Sarah also struggles with the sensory environment. The constant ringing of the phones and the bright fluorescent lights leave her feeling drained and irritable by the end of the day. She often has meltdowns when she gets home.

Sarah is an excellent midwife. But the environment is failing her.

## The ADHD midwife

**Strengths:**

- **Crisis management:** ADHDers often thrive in high-pressure situations. They can remain calm and focused during emergencies, thanks to their ability to hyperfocus under stress.

- **Creativity and innovation:** ADHD midwives are often creative thinkers who can come up with novel solutions to complex problems. They are often the ones driving quality improvement projects.

- **Energy and enthusiasm:** ADHDers often bring a high level of energy and enthusiasm to their work. They can be highly motivating and engaging with patients and colleagues.

- **Adaptability:** ADHD midwives are often flexible and adaptable, able to switch tasks quickly and respond to changing situations.

- **Rapport building:** ADHDers can be highly charismatic and skilled at building rapport with patients. They often have a great sense of humor and a warm, approachable manner.

**Challenges:**

- **Distractibility:** The constant interruptions and competing demands of a busy maternity unit can make it difficult to focus. This can lead to errors and omissions.

- **Time management:** Difficulty with time management and organization can lead to missed deadlines, late arrivals, and chaotic workflows.

- **Impulsivity:** Impulsive decision-making can be risky in a clinical setting. ADHD midwives may struggle with interrupting others or speaking without thinking.

- **Emotional dysregulation:** ADHDers often experience emotions intensely. They may struggle with frustration tolerance, rejection sensitivity, and mood swings.

- **Boredom and under-stimulation:** While ADHDers thrive in fast-paced environments, they can also struggle with boredom during quiet periods or repetitive tasks. This can lead to restlessness and procrastination.

**Case Example: David, the ADHD Midwife**

David is a community midwife. He is beloved by his patients for his warm personality and his ability to make them feel at ease. He is also a creative problem-solver, always coming up with new ways to support families.

But David struggles with organization. His car is a mess, his paperwork is always behind, and he often runs late for appointments. He relies on reminders and checklists to keep him on track, but even then, things slip through the cracks.

David also struggles with emotional regulation. He takes criticism personally and can become defensive when challenged. He often feels overwhelmed by the administrative demands of the job.

David is a compassionate and skilled midwife. But the organizational demands of the job are overwhelming him.

## The importance of reasonable adjustments

Both Sarah and David have the potential to be exceptional midwives. But they need the right support and accommodations to thrive.

The concept of "reasonable adjustments" is key here. Under equality legislation in many countries, employers have a legal duty to provide reasonable adjustments for disabled employees, including those who are neurodivergent.

Reasonable adjustments are changes to the work environment or work practices that enable a person to perform their job effectively. They are not about giving someone an unfair advantage; they are about leveling the playing field.

What might reasonable adjustments look like for neurodivergent midwives?

### Sensory adjustments:

- Providing a quiet workspace for documentation and breaks.
- Allowing the use of noise-canceling headphones or earplugs.
- Adjusting the lighting in clinical areas.
- Minimizing strong smells by using scent-free cleaning products.

### Communication adjustments:

- Providing written instructions and agendas for meetings.
- Using clear, direct communication styles.
- Offering regular feedback and check-ins.
- Providing mentorship and coaching on communication skills.

**Organizational adjustments:**

- Providing assistive technology, such as speech-to-text software or digital organizers.
- Offering flexible working arrangements, such as annualized hours or compressed shifts.
- Providing support with planning and prioritization.
- Breaking down large tasks into smaller, manageable steps.

**Social adjustments:**

- Providing clear expectations about social interactions at work.
- Creating opportunities for structured social activities, rather than relying on informal networking.
- Promoting a culture of psychological safety, where people feel safe to speak up and ask for help.

The key is that adjustments must be individualized. What works for one Autistic midwife might not work for another. The process should be collaborative, involving the midwife, their manager, and occupational health.

### Strategies for self-care and avoiding professional burnout

Midwifery is a demanding profession. Burnout rates are high across the board. But for neurodivergent midwives, the risk of burnout is even higher.

The constant sensory overload, the emotional intensity of the work, the pressure to mask and conform—it all takes a toll. Neurodivergent people often experience "Autistic burnout" or "ADHD burnout," which is a state of profound physical and mental exhaustion caused by chronic stress and the cumulative burden of navigating a world not built for them (Raymaker et al., 2020).

Self-care is not a luxury; it is a necessity. It is about putting on your own oxygen mask first so you can continue to help others.

But traditional self-care advice (like bubble baths and yoga) often falls short for neurodivergent people. We need strategies that are tailored to our unique needs and challenges.

## Understanding your sensory profile

The first step is to understand your own sensory profile. What are your triggers? What helps you regulate?

Conduct a sensory audit of your work environment. Identify the hotspots for sensory overload. Can you make any adjustments? Can you use sensory tools to help you cope?

Incorporate sensory breaks into your day. Even a few minutes in a quiet room or a walk outside can make a difference.

## Managing energy levels

Neurodivergent people often have fluctuating energy levels. We need to learn to work with our energy, rather than against it.

The "Spoons Theory" is a helpful metaphor here. It suggests that we all start the day with a certain number of "spoons" (units of energy). Every task, every interaction, every sensory input uses up spoons. Neurodivergent people often have fewer spoons to begin with, and they use them up faster.

Track your energy levels throughout the day. Identify the activities that drain you and the ones that replenish you. Try to balance your workload accordingly.

Be realistic about what you can achieve. It is okay to say no. It is okay to ask for help.

## Developing executive function skills

Executive dysfunction is a common challenge for neurodivergent midwives. We need strategies to support our planning, organization, and time management.

- **Externalize information:** Get everything out of your head and onto paper or a digital organizer. Use checklists, reminders, and calendars.

- **Break it down:** Break down large tasks into small, manageable steps.

- **Use visual aids:** Use color-coding, mind maps, and flowcharts to organize information.

- **Establish routines:** Routines can help automate tasks and reduce cognitive load.

- **Body doubling:** Working alongside another person, even if you are working on different tasks, can help improve focus and motivation.

## Building a support network

Connection is key to preventing burnout. We need people who understand us, support us, and advocate for us.

Connect with other neurodivergent midwives. Peer support groups can be incredibly validating. They provide a safe space to share experiences, exchange strategies, and celebrate successes.

Seek out mentorship from senior midwives who are neuro-affirming and supportive.

Build a support network outside of work too. Friends, family, therapists, and coaches can provide valuable perspective and support.

## Practicing self-compassion

This is perhaps the most important strategy of all. We need to learn to be kind to ourselves.

We live in a world that constantly tells us we are "too much" or "not enough." We internalize these messages and become our own harshest critics.

Self-compassion involves treating ourselves with the same kindness, understanding, and acceptance that we would offer a friend.

Acknowledge your challenges without judgment. Celebrate your strengths. Forgive yourself for your mistakes.

Remember that you are not broken. You are different. And different is good.

## The future of the neurodivergent midwife

The future of midwifery depends on our ability to embrace diversity in all its forms. This includes neurodiversity.

We need to move beyond awareness and acceptance towards genuine inclusion and celebration.

We need to create a profession where neurodivergent midwives are not just surviving, but thriving.

When we support neurodivergent midwives, we create a more compassionate, innovative, and resilient workforce. We also improve the quality of care we provide to neurodivergent families. Neurodivergent midwives often have a unique ability to connect with and advocate for neurodivergent patients. They understand the challenges firsthand.

The path forward requires systemic change. It requires organizations to invest in training, resources, and accommodations. It requires leaders to champion neuro-inclusive practices.

But it also requires individual action. It requires us to challenge our own biases, educate ourselves about neurodiversity, and support our neurodivergent colleagues.

It is time to bring neurodiversity out of the shadows and into the light. It is time to recognize the incredible contributions of neurodivergent midwives. And it is time to build a profession where everyone feels safe, valued, and empowered to be their authentic selves.

---

**Key Takeaways**

- Neurodivergent midwives bring unique strengths to the profession, including attention to detail, creativity, empathy, and crisis management skills.

- They also face significant challenges, including sensory overload, communication differences, executive dysfunction, and emotional dysregulation.

- Acknowledging neurodiversity and creating a culture of disclosure are essential first steps towards inclusion.

- Reasonable adjustments are crucial for enabling neurodivergent midwives to thrive. These adjustments should be individualized and collaborative.

- Self-care strategies tailored to neurodivergent needs are essential for preventing burnout.

- Strategies include understanding your sensory profile, managing energy levels, developing executive function skills, building a support network, and practicing self-compassion.

- Supporting neurodivergent midwives leads to a more compassionate, innovative, and resilient profession.

## The Path to Truly Inclusive Care

We have covered a lot of ground together. From understanding the basics of neurodiversity to implementing systemic change. From supporting Autistic parents during labor to advocating for neurodivergent midwives.

The journey towards inclusive midwifery is complex. It is challenging. And it is absolutely necessary.

This is not just about improving patient satisfaction scores or reducing complaints. It is about upholding fundamental human rights. It is about ensuring that every person, regardless of their neurotype, has access to safe, respectful, and affirming perinatal care.

The strategies we have discussed are not just theoretical concepts. They are practical tools that you can use to make a real difference in the lives of neurodivergent families.

**Summary of key strategies**

Let's briefly revisit the core strategies that underpin inclusive midwifery.

1. **Education and Awareness:** Understanding the diversity of neurodivergent experiences is the foundation. This means moving beyond stereotypes and embracing a neuro-affirming approach. It means ongoing training for all staff, ideally led by neurodivergent individuals.

2. **Communication Adjustments:** Clear, literal, and patient communication is essential. This includes providing written information, using visual aids, and respecting different communication styles. It means asking people how they prefer to communicate and honoring their preferences.

3. **Sensory Accommodations:** The perinatal environment is often sensory-overwhelming. We must create low-stimulus spaces, offer sensory toolkits, and minimize unnecessary noise and light. We must proactively ask about sensory needs and make adjustments accordingly.

4. **Individualized Care Planning:** Standardized protocols do not work for everyone. We need flexible, individualized care plans that are co-created with the neurodivergent person. This includes birth preferences, communication passports, and sensory passports.

5. **Continuity of Carer:** Building trust and rapport is crucial for neurodivergent people. Continuity of carer models provide consistency and reduce anxiety.

6. **Advocacy and Empowerment:** We must empower neurodivergent people to advocate for their own needs and preferences. This means providing information, supporting decision-making, and respecting bodily autonomy.

7. **Systemic Change:** Individual efforts are not enough. We need systemic change to ensure that inclusive care is the default. This includes developing departmental guidelines, appointing Neurodiversity Leads, and creating supportive policies.

8. **Supporting Neurodivergent Staff:** Inclusive care extends to the workforce. We must acknowledge and support neurodivergent midwives, providing reasonable adjustments and fostering a culture of psychological safety.

## The lasting impact of affirming care

The impact of affirming care cannot be overstated. When a neurodivergent person feels seen, heard, and respected during their perinatal journey, the effects ripple outwards.

It reduces the risk of birth trauma. Traumatic birth experiences are unfortunately common among neurodivergent people. Affirming care can help prevent trauma by promoting safety, control, and dignity.

It improves perinatal mental health. Neurodivergent people are at higher risk of anxiety, depression, and PTSD during the perinatal period. Affirming care provides a buffer against these challenges by reducing stress and promoting well-being.

It strengthens the parent-infant bond. When parents feel supported and empowered, they are better able to bond with their babies. Affirming care promotes a positive transition to parenthood.

It fosters trust in the healthcare system. Many neurodivergent people have experienced discrimination and misunderstanding in healthcare settings. Affirming care can help repair this mistrust and encourage engagement with services.

The impact extends beyond the individual family. When we provide inclusive care, we challenge societal stigma and discrimination. We promote a more compassionate and equitable world.

## A final call to action for all midwives

You have the power to make a difference. Every interaction, every decision, every action you take matters.

You do not need to be an expert on neurodiversity to provide inclusive care. You just need to be curious, compassionate, and committed to learning.

Start small. Start where you are.

Here is my challenge to you:

1. **Educate yourself:** Read books, articles, and blogs written by neurodivergent people. Listen to podcasts. Attend workshops. Keep learning.

2. **Reflect on your practice:** Examine your own biases and assumptions. How might they be affecting your interactions with neurodivergent patients and colleagues?

3. **Make one change:** Choose one thing you can do differently this week. Maybe it is adjusting the lighting in your clinic room. Maybe it is offering written information proactively. Maybe it is simply asking, "How can I best support you today?"

4. **Advocate for change:** Use your voice to advocate for systemic change within your organization. Start conversations about neurodiversity. Share your successes. Challenge discriminatory practices.

5. **Support your colleagues:** Be an ally to your neurodivergent colleagues. Offer support, understanding, and compassion.

The path to inclusive midwifery is a journey, not a destination. There will be challenges and setbacks along the way. But the work is worth doing.

By embracing neurodiversity and championing inclusive care, we can transform maternity services. We can create a future where every birth is a safe, empowering, and joyous experience for all.

Thank you for joining me on this journey. Now, go out there and make a difference.

# Appendix A: Neuro-Affirming Birth Plan/Access Document Template

Let's talk about birth plans. You've probably seen those standard templates online. They usually focus on things like, "I want delayed cord clamping" or "I prefer intermittent monitoring." And look, those things are good to know. But here's the issue. Those plans often fall apart when things get intense. Why? Because they are based on *preferences* for a physiological event, not *requirements* for accessibility.

For neurodivergent folks, a standard birth plan often misses the mark entirely. It doesn't explain *how* you process information, *how* your environment affects you, or *what* support you need just to stay regulated.

So, we're ditching the traditional "birth plan." Instead, we are creating an **Access Document**.

This is different. An Access Document is a tool for communication. It clearly states your needs so your birth team can provide safe, equitable, and affirming care. It's not a list of demands. It's a guide on how to work with your unique brain and body. Think of this document as your user manual.

**How to use this template**

Below is a template you can copy and adapt. Be specific. The more detail you provide, the better your team can support you.

1. **Fill it out when you are calm.** Seriously, don't wait until you're stressed or close to your due date. Do it now.

2. **Keep it brief.** Aim for one to two pages maximum. Use bullet points. Your nurses and providers are busy; they need the information quickly.

3. **Discuss it beforehand.** Review this document with your provider (midwife or obstetrician) during a prenatal appointment, maybe around 34-36 weeks. Ask them to place a copy in your official medical file.

4. **Bring copies.** Have several printed copies in your hospital bag. When you arrive, hand one to the triage nurse, one to your labor nurse, and tape one up on the wall in your birth room where everyone can see it.

This is about making your birth experience accessible. You deserve that.

---

## MY BIRTH ACCESS DOCUMENT

My Name: [Your Name]

My Pronouns: [e.g., she/her, they/them]

My Due Date: [Date]

My Support People: [Name(s) and relationship(s), e.g., Partner, Doula]

My Provider: [Name of Midwife or OB]

### About Me and My Access Needs

*Please read this carefully. This document explains my access needs to help you provide safe and affirming care during my birth experience.*

I identify as [e.g., Autistic, ADHDer, Neurodivergent]. This means my brain works differently. I may process information, communicate, and experience sensory input in ways you are not used to.

### Key things to know about me:

- [e.g., I process information literally and logically. Abstract concepts are confusing.]

- [e.g., I have high sensory sensitivity, especially to sound and bright light. These cause me physical discomfort.]

- [e.g., I may not make typical eye contact. This does not mean I am not listening or engaged.]

- [e.g., When stressed or overwhelmed, I may shut down and become non-speaking or minimally speaking.]

- [e.g., I use stimming (self-stimulatory behavior) like rocking or hand-flapping to stay calm. This is necessary for me. Please do not interfere with this.]

- [e.g., I struggle with interoception (sensing internal body signals) and may not recognize pain or the urge to push clearly.]

## Communication Preferences

*My ability to communicate will likely change during labor, especially when I am in pain or tired.*

### Please DO:

- **Speak directly to me**, not just my support person.

- Use **clear, literal, and concise language**. Avoid metaphors or vague terms (e.g., say "needle stick" instead of "little pinch").

- Give me **extra time to process** information and respond. Wait silently for at least 10 seconds.

- **Write things down** or use visual aids if I am having trouble understanding spoken words.

- Ask **one question at a time**. Wait for my answer before asking the next.

- **Explain what you are doing before you do it.** Announce when you are entering or leaving the room.

- If I become non-speaking, use my backup communication method: [e.g., text-to-speech app on my phone, whiteboard, specific hand gestures (thumbs up/down)].

## Please AVOID:

- Asking open-ended questions like "How are you feeling?" Ask specific questions instead.

- Using phrases like "Just relax" or "Calm down." (This is counterproductive).

- Whispering or having non-essential conversations in the room.

- Assuming my needs based on my facial expressions (I may not express pain typically).

- Rushing me to make decisions unless it is a life-threatening emergency.

## Sensory Environment

*Creating a low-sensory environment is crucial for my regulation and ability to cope with labor.*

## Lighting:

- Keep lights **dimmed or off**. Use natural light if available.

- I will bring [e.g., battery-operated fairy lights, eye mask, sunglasses].

- Minimize flashing lights on equipment. Turn screens away from me if possible.

## Sound:

- Keep the room **as quiet as possible**. Speak in soft, calm voices.

- Minimize beeping from monitors. Reduce the volume if safe to do so.

- Close the door fully.

- I will use [e.g., noise-canceling headphones, ear defenders, white noise machine].

## Touch and Physical Contact:

- **Ask for consent before every touch**, even for routine checks. This is non-negotiable.

- Explain exactly where and how you will touch me before you do it.

- I prefer [e.g., firm pressure, light touch, no touch at all].

- Cervical exams are very distressing/triggering for me. Please limit them to what is absolutely medically necessary and use trauma-informed techniques (e.g., use extra lubrication, allow me to choose the position, stop immediately if I ask).

## Smell:

- Please avoid wearing strong perfumes, lotions, or scented deodorant.

- Minimize strong clinical smells (like cleaning products) if possible.

- I will bring [e.g., preferred essential oils on a cotton ball] for comfort.

## During Labor and Birth

## Monitoring:

- I prefer [e.g., intermittent monitoring with a handheld doppler, continuous external monitoring].

- If continuous monitoring is needed, the feeling of the belts is difficult for me. I may need [e.g., wireless monitoring, frequent breaks, a soft cloth placed underneath the bands].

## Movement and Coping:

- I need freedom of movement. Do not ask me to stay in bed unless medically required.

- I will use these coping tools: [e.g., stimming, vocalizing (humming/groaning), TENS unit, bath/shower, birth ball].

- My pain expression might look like [e.g., silence and withdrawal, humming, intense focus]. Do not assume I am coping well just because I am quiet.

**Pushing Stage:**

- I may need explicit, step-by-step guidance on how to push due to difficulties with proprioception (body awareness).

- Please avoid shouting or enthusiastic "cheerleading." Calm, clear instructions are best.

- I prefer to push instinctively in the position that feels right for me [e.g., side-lying, hands and knees].

**If a Cesarean Birth is Needed**

*A change in plans can be very dysregulating. Clear communication is essential.*

- Explain the reason for the Cesarean clearly and logically.

- Provide a step-by-step overview of what will happen.

- Allow my support person [Name] to stay with me at all times.

- **In the Operating Room:**
  - Minimize noise and non-essential conversation.
  - Explain sensations before they happen (e.g., "You will feel pressure now").
  - Allow me to wear noise-canceling headphones or listen to music.
  - If possible, use a clear drape or lower the drape so I can see the baby.

- o Place the baby skin-to-skin as soon as possible.

## Immediate Postpartum and Baby Care

*The time immediately after birth can be overwhelming. I need support to bond and recover.*

- Prioritize the "golden hour" for uninterrupted skin-to-skin contact.

- Delay non-urgent newborn procedures until after the first feed.

- Explain all procedures (e.g., fundal massage, sutures) before doing them. Consent is still required.

- **Feeding:** I plan to [e.g., breastfeed/chestfeed, formula feed, combination feed]. I may need extra support with positioning and latch due to sensory sensitivities or motor coordination challenges.

- Please direct all questions about the baby to me or my partner.

**Thank you for supporting me and respecting my access needs.**

# Appendix B: Environmental Sensory Audit Checklist

Hospitals and birth centers? Let's be honest. They are often sensory nightmares. Think about it. The bright fluorescent lights that buzz, the constant beeping of machines, the strong smells of cleaning solutions, the unfamiliar textures of those scratchy hospital gowns. For someone with sensory processing differences, this environment isn't just uncomfortable. It can be actively harmful.

It can increase stress, amplify pain perception, and make it much harder to cope with labor

This checklist is designed to help you audit your intended birth environment and identify potential sensory triggers. If you are planning a hospital or birth center birth, try to do this during a tour. If a tour isn't possible (sometimes they aren't), you can use this checklist when you first arrive in your labor room to make quick adjustments.

Your goal is to create a "sensory safe zone." A space where your nervous system can feel secure.

### How to use this checklist

Go through each sensory category. Identify the potential issues. Then, brainstorm solutions. What can you remove, reduce, or introduce to make the space work for you? We are looking at the eight sensory systems here, not just the standard five.

### SENSORY AUDIT CHECKLIST

### 1. Sight (Visual Input)

Bright lights, clutter, and flashing monitors can be visually overwhelming and stressful.

**Audit Questions:**

- Are the main lights fluorescent? Are they bright? Do they flicker or buzz?

- Can the lights be dimmed? Can they be turned off completely?

- Is there natural light? Can the blinds or curtains be adjusted easily?

- Are there flashing lights on the monitors (IV pump, EFM)?

- Can the screens be turned away from my line of sight or dimmed?

- Is the room cluttered with medical equipment? Is there a lot of "visual noise"?

**Action Plan Ideas:**

- Ask the nurse to dim or turn off overhead lights immediately upon arrival.

- Bring an eye mask or sunglasses (yes, indoors, it helps).

- Bring alternative lighting (battery-operated candles, fairy lights) to create a calm ambiance.

- Ask if flashing indicators can be minimized or covered with tape if safe.

- Cover distracting equipment or busy patterns with a familiar blanket or towel.

- Hang up affirming visual anchors (photos, affirmation cards).

## 2. Sound (Auditory Input)

Hospitals are loud. Unpredictable noises are especially jarring to the nervous system.

**Audit Questions:**

- How loud is the hallway noise (talking, carts rolling, phones ringing)?
- Does the door close completely? Is there a gap underneath?
- How loud are the monitor beeps and alarms? Can the volume be adjusted?
- Is the air conditioning or heating unit noisy or rattling?
- Is there unnecessary chatter in the room by staff?

**Action Plan Ideas:**

- Keep the door closed. Place a rolled-up towel at the base of the door to block sound.
- Put a sign on the door asking for staff to knock gently and speak softly.
- Ask staff to reduce monitor volumes if medically safe.
- Request that staff avoid non-essential conversations in the room.
- Use noise-canceling headphones or high-fidelity earplugs.
- Play preferred sounds (calming music, brown noise, nature sounds) using a portable speaker.

### 3. Smell (Olfactory Input)

Smells can be intense and triggering, especially with pregnancy-heightened senses.

**Audit Questions:**

- Are there strong smells of cleaning products or antiseptics?
- Are staff wearing perfume, scented lotion, or strong deodorant? (This is a big one.)
- Are there strong food smells coming from the cafeteria or staff break room?

- Is the room stuffy or poorly ventilated?

**Action Plan Ideas:**

- Request that staff attending you avoid wearing scented products (include this in your Access Document).

- Use preferred scents for comfort (e.g., lavender, peppermint, or just the smell of a familiar pillowcase from home) on a cotton ball near you.

- If a smell is bothering you, ask if the source can be removed (e.g., taking out the trash promptly).

- Use a portable fan for better air circulation.

### 4. Touch (Tactile Input)

Unfamiliar textures and unwanted touch can be highly dysregulating, even painful.

**Audit Questions:**

- What is the texture of the hospital gown and bedding? Is it scratchy, stiff, or papery?

- Are the EFM belts tight, itchy, or uncomfortable?

- Is the room temperature too hot or too cold? Can it be controlled?

- Are IV lines or blood pressure cuffs irritating the skin?

**Action Plan Ideas:**

- Bring your own comfortable clothing to labor in (a soft nightgown, robe, large t-shirt).

- Bring your own bedding (pillows, blankets) from home.

- If continuous monitoring is needed, ask about wireless options or request a soft fabric barrier underneath the bands.

- Ask for adjustments to the room temperature. Bring socks and a favorite cardigan.

- Use preferred tactile stim tools (fidget spinners, stress balls, soft fabrics).

- Clearly communicate your preferences for touch (firm vs. light) and the absolute need for consent before any physical contact.

## 5. Taste (Gustatory Input)

Hospital food and restrictions on eating can be difficult, especially if you rely on "safe foods."

### Audit Questions:

- What are the policies on eating and drinking during labor?

- What kind of fluids are provided (water, juice, broth)?

- Is the taste or texture of the provided drinks acceptable?

### Action Plan Ideas:

- Discuss eating and drinking policies with your provider beforehand.

- Bring your own preferred snacks and drinks (if allowed). Focus on foods that are easy to digest and comforting.

- Bring reusable straws (sometimes the texture of the hospital straws is just... wrong) or preferred cups.

- Have hard candies or lollipops available for dry mouth and energy.

## 6. Movement (Vestibular Input)

This relates to balance and spatial orientation. Being forced to stay still can be very stressful.

### Audit Questions:

- Is there enough space to move around, rock, sway, or change positions?

- Are there restrictions on movement (e.g., being confined to bed due to monitoring or IV)?

- Are there tools available to support movement (birth ball, rocking chair)?

**Action Plan Ideas:**

- Keep the floor space clear of obstacles.

- Request wireless monitoring or intermittent monitoring to allow for movement.

- Use the shower or bath, as the buoyancy of water supports movement.

## 7. Body Awareness (Proprioceptive Input)

This is knowing where your body is in space. Deep pressure and "heavy work" are often regulating.

**Audit Questions:**

- Is there access to deep pressure (e.g., massage, counter-pressure)?

- Are weighted blankets allowed?

- Are there tools for resistance (e.g., a rebozo or sheet to pull on)?

**Action Plan Ideas:**

- Train your support person in counter-pressure techniques for contractions.

- Bring a weighted blanket for use during rest periods or postpartum.

- Use compression socks.

## 8. Internal Sensations (Interoceptive Input)

This is the ability to sense internal signals like hunger, thirst, pain, and the need to use the bathroom. It's easy to lose touch with these when you're stressed.

**Audit Questions:**

- Will I be reminded to eat and drink?
- Will I be encouraged to use the bathroom regularly?
- Are my descriptions of pain or sensation respected?

**Action Plan Ideas:**

- Set a timer on your phone or ask your partner to remind you to sip water every 15 minutes.
- Plan to try to use the bathroom every 1-2 hours.
- Use descriptive language or a numerical scale to communicate pain levels clearly.

# Appendix C: Quick-Reference Communication Guide (Do's and Don'ts)

Communication during birth is everything. It's how you express your needs, how you receive information, and how you make decisions. But here's the deal: what works for most people might not work for a neurodivergent person, especially when they are under stress.

During labor, the brain changes. The thinking part of the brain (the prefrontal cortex) gets quieter, and the instinctual part takes over. For autistic people, ADHDers, and others, this shift can make communication even harder. They might experience shutdowns, become non-speaking (situational mutism), or struggle to process spoken language (Moore, 2016).

This guide is for your birth team: your nurses, midwife, obstetrician, doula, and yes, even your partner. It's a quick reference on how to communicate in a way that is clear, respectful, and affirming.

Share this guide. Talk about it. Make sure everyone understands that *how* they speak to you is just as important as *what* they say.

---

## QUICK-REFERENCE COMMUNICATION GUIDE FOR SUPPORTING NEURODIVERGENT PARENTS

**The Goal:** To ensure clear communication, reduce anxiety, and support informed decision-making. Assume competence. Always.

**Understanding the Context:**

- Neurodivergent individuals (e.g., Autistic, ADHD) process information and communicate differently.

- Stress, pain, and sensory overload during labor significantly impact communication abilities.

- They may become minimally speaking or non-speaking when overwhelmed (shutdown).

- They may not express pain or emotions in typical ways (alexithymia).

## PLEASE DO (Affirming Communication)

### 1. Be Clear and Direct

- **DO** use concrete, literal language. Say exactly what you mean.

    - *Instead of:* "I'm just going to pop this cuff on."

    - *Try:* "I am going to wrap this cuff around your arm to check your blood pressure. It will feel tight."

- **DO** give information in small chunks.

- **DO** ask one question at a time. Wait patiently for a response before moving on.

### 2. Allow Processing Time

- **DO** allow extra time (at least 10 seconds) for processing and responding. Silence does not mean they haven't heard you. Don't fill the silence with more words.

- **DO** check for understanding.

    - *Try:* "Can you tell me what we decided so I know we are on the same page?"

### 3. Respect Communication Differences

- **DO** speak directly to the birthing person, not just their partner or doula.

- **DO** recognize that lack of eye contact does not mean lack of attention or respect. It often helps with listening.

- **DO** use alternative communication methods if they become non-speaking (whiteboard, text-to-speech app, hand signals). Plan this in advance.

## 4. Provide Predictability and Consent

- **DO** explain what you are going to do before you do it, every single time.

- **DO** announce when you are entering or leaving the room.

- **DO** ask for consent before any touch or procedure. Wait for a clear "yes." If they say "stop," stop immediately.

## 5. Support Regulation

- **DO** help maintain a low-sensory environment (quiet voices, dimmed lights).

- **DO** respect self-regulatory behaviors (stimming, rocking, humming). These are essential coping mechanisms, not behaviors to be stopped.

- **DO** offer reassurance using facts and logic, rather than emotional appeals.

## PLEASE AVOID (Barriers to Communication)

## 1. Avoid Vague Language and Assumptions

- **AVOID** metaphors, sarcasm, euphemisms, or vague instructions.

   - *Instead of:* "Listen to your body."

   - *Try:* "Tell me if you feel pressure in your bottom."

- **AVOID** assuming needs based on facial expressions or tone of voice.

- **AVOID** open-ended questions like "How are you feeling?"

## 2. Avoid Rushing and Pressure

- **AVOID** rushing the person to make decisions (unless it is an immediate emergency).

- **AVOID** interrupting or talking over them.

- **AVOID** asking repetitive questions if they haven't answered yet. Rephrase if necessary, but first, just wait.

## 3. Avoid Dismissing Concerns

- **AVOID** minimizing their experience or sensory sensitivities. (e.g., "That noise isn't that loud.")

- **AVOID** phrases like "Just relax," "Calm down," or "It's not that bad." This is invalidating and unhelpful.

- **AVOID** reacting negatively to meltdowns or shutdowns. These are signs of extreme distress, not behavioral problems.

## 4. Avoid Sensory Overload

- **AVOID** unnecessary chatter, whispering, or loud noises in the room.

- **AVOID** strong scents (perfume, scented lotions).

- **AVOID** unnecessary physical contact or sudden movements.

## In an Emergency

If rapid action is needed, communication must be even clearer. Do not panic.

- **Use the person's name.**

- **State the problem clearly:** "The baby's heart rate is low."

- **State the required action:** "We need you to turn onto your left side right now."

- **Provide brief, logical reassurance:** "This position helps get more oxygen to the baby."

# Appendix D: Glossary of Neurodiversity-Affirming Terms

Words matter. They really do. The language we use shapes how we think about ourselves and how others perceive us. For a long time, the language used to describe neurodivergence (like autism or ADHD) has been based on a medical model. It focused on deficits, disorders, and impairments. It implied something was broken and needed fixing.

We are moving away from that. We are embracing the **neurodiversity paradigm**. This perspective recognizes that differences in brain function are natural variations of the human experience (Walker, 2021).

This glossary defines key terms using affirming language. It's about understanding the concepts without the baggage of pathologizing labels. Using this language can help you advocate for yourself and connect with others who share your experiences.

A quick note on preference: Language is personal. While many Autistic adults prefer identity-first language ("Autistic person"), some prefer person-first language ("person with autism") (Kenny et al., 2016). Always respect the individual's preference.

## GLOSSARY OF TERMS

**Ableism:** Discrimination and prejudice against people with disabilities. It is the belief that "typical" abilities are superior and that disabled people are inferior or need to be fixed.

**Access Needs:** The specific requirements a person has to fully participate in an environment, activity, or conversation. We prefer this term over "special needs." Everyone has access needs.

**Alexithymia:** Difficulty identifying, describing, and understanding one's own emotions and internal states. It's not that the feelings aren't there; it's that the connection between the feeling and the words is fuzzy. This can make recognizing labor sensations challenging.

**Autistic Burnout:** A state of intense physical, mental, and emotional exhaustion. It often results from long-term masking, sensory overload, and the chronic stress of living in a world not designed for autistic needs. It can lead to a loss of skills and reduced tolerance for stimuli (Raymaker et al., 2020).

**Co-regulation:** A supportive process where one person's calm nervous system helps to soothe and regulate another person's distressed nervous system. In birth, this is often the role of the partner or doula.

**Double Empathy Problem:** A theory suggesting that communication breakdowns between Autistic and non-Autistic people are a two-way street. It's not just that Autistic people struggle to understand neurotypicals; neurotypicals also struggle to understand Autistic perspectives and communication styles (Milton, 2012).

**Echolalia:** The repetition of words, phrases, or sounds spoken by others. This is a valid form of communication and self-regulation, not meaningless repetition.

**Executive Function:** A set of mental skills that help us get things done. These include working memory, flexible thinking, planning, organization, time management, and self-control. Many neurodivergent people experience challenges with executive function.

**Hyperfocus:** An intense state of concentration on a specific task or topic, often to the exclusion of everything else. While it can be a strength, it can also make switching attention difficult.

**Interoception:** The sense that helps us understand and feel what's going on inside our bodies. It includes recognizing hunger, thirst, temperature, pain, and emotions.

**Masking (or Camouflaging):** The conscious or unconscious suppression of natural neurodivergent traits to appear neurotypical. This includes suppressing stims, mimicking social behaviors, or scripting conversations. Masking takes significant energy and leads to burnout.

**Meltdown:** An intense, involuntary reaction to overwhelming stress, sensory input, or emotional distress. It is a sign of extreme overload. Meltdowns are not tantrums; the person has lost control and needs support and safety.

**Neurodivergent (ND):** An umbrella term for people whose brains function differently from what is considered typical or "normal." This includes Autistic people, ADHDers, dyslexics, and those with dyspraxia, among others.

**Neurodiversity:** The diversity of human brains and minds. It refers to the natural variation in neurological function within the human species.

**Neuro-Affirming Care:** An approach to care that respects and validates the individual's neurodivergent identity. It focuses on strengths, accommodates access needs, and supports the person's well-being without trying to "fix" their neurodivergence.

**Neurotypical (NT):** A person whose brain function aligns with the dominant societal standards of "normal."

**Proprioception:** The sense of body awareness. It tells us where our body parts are in space and how they are moving.

**Rejection Sensitive Dysphoria (RSD):** Extreme emotional sensitivity and pain triggered by the perception—real or imagined—of being rejected, teased, or criticized. It is common among ADHDers.

**Sensory Overload:** When the sensory input from the environment exceeds the brain's capacity to process it, leading to stress, confusion, and distress.

**Shutdown:** A response to overwhelm where the person withdraws, becomes quiet, and may be unable to communicate (situational mutism) or move. It is a protective mechanism against overload, often less visible than a meltdown.

**Situational Mutism (Sometimes called Selective Mutism):** An inability to speak in specific situations, often due to high stress, anxiety, or overwhelm. It is not a choice.

**Stimming (Self-Stimulatory Behavior):** Repetitive movements, sounds, or actions that help regulate the nervous system, express emotions, or cope with sensory input. Examples include hand-flapping, rocking, humming, repeating phrases, or manipulating objects. Stimming is healthy and necessary.

# Appendix E: Resources and Organizations

Finding your people is so important. When you are navigating pregnancy, birth, and parenthood as a neurodivergent person, it can feel incredibly isolating. You might feel like no one understands your experiences or your needs.

But you are definitely not alone. There is a growing community of neurodivergent parents and professionals who get it. They are advocating for change, sharing resources, and supporting each other.

This list includes organizations, websites, and support groups in the UK and internationally. It's not exhaustive, but it's a good starting point. Reach out. Connect. Find the support you deserve.

## UNITED KINGDOM (UK) RESOURCES

### Maternity and Neurodiversity Advocacy

- **Autistic Parents UK:** A user-led organization providing support, information, and advocacy for autistic parents. They offer peer support groups and resources tailored to the autistic parenting experience.

- **Maternity Action:** Provides free advice and information on rights at work, benefits, and maternity care for pregnant women and new parents. They have resources on discrimination and accessing support.

- **Birthrights:** The UK charity dedicated to protecting human rights in childbirth. They provide advice on legal rights and advocate for respectful maternity care. If you feel your rights have been violated, Birthrights can be a valuable resource.

- **AIMS (Association for Improvements in the Maternity Services):** Provides independent support and information about maternity choices. They offer a helpline and resources on navigating the maternity system.

- **Maternity Autism Research Group (MARG):** A collaboration of researchers, clinicians, and autistic people focused on improving maternity care for autistic individuals.

## Neurodiversity Organizations (General)

- **National Autistic Society (NAS):** The leading UK charity for autistic people and their families. They provide information, support, and campaign for a society that works for autistic people.

- **ADHD Foundation:** Works to improve the emotional well-being and organizational outcomes for people with ADHD, autism, dyslexia, dyspraxia, and other neurodevelopmental conditions.

- **The Donaldson Trust:** A Scottish organization focused on neurodiversity, advocating for a neuro-inclusive society.

## Mental Health Support

- **PANDAS Foundation:** Provides support and advice for parents experiencing perinatal mental illness, including postnatal depression and anxiety.

- **Mind:** A mental health charity providing advice and support to anyone experiencing a mental health problem, with information on perinatal mental health.

## INTERNATIONAL RESOURCES

## Maternity and Neurodiversity Advocacy

- **Autistic Women & Nonbinary Network (AWN) (USA):** Provides community, support, and resources for autistic women, girls, nonbinary people, and all others of marginalized genders.

- **The Autistic Self Advocacy Network (ASAN) (USA/International):** A nonprofit organization run by and for autistic people. ASAN advocates for policies that improve the lives of autistic people. Their motto is "Nothing About Us Without Us."

- **Reframing Autism (Australia):** Run by Autistic people, providing information and resources grounded in the lived experience of Autism, promoting a neurodiversity-affirming perspective.

## Neurodiversity Organizations (General)

- **CHADD (Children and Adults with Attention-Deficit/Hyperactivity Disorder) (USA):** Provides support, training, and advocacy for people with ADHD and their families.

- **Yellow Ladybugs (Australia):** An organization dedicated to the happiness, success, and celebration of autistic girls, women, and gender-diverse individuals.

## Perinatal Support and Education

- **Postpartum Support International (PSI) (International):** The world's leading organization dedicated to helping people suffering from perinatal mood disorders. They offer a helpline, resources, and connections to local support providers.

- **Evidence Based Birth (USA/Global):** Provides accessible, evidence-based information on birth practices. While not specifically neurodiversity-focused, their resources on consent and patient advocacy are highly valuable.

## Books

- *Unmasking Autism: Discovering the New Faces of Neurodiversity* by Devon Price, PhD.

- *Divergent Mind: Thriving in a World That Wasn't Designed for You* by Jenara Nerenberg.

- *Neuroqueer Heresies* by Nick Walker.

- *The Reason I Jump* by Naoki Higashida.

- *The Autistic Advocate's Guide to an Affirming Pregnancy and Birth* by Terra Vance.

---

## Putting Your Tools to Work

These appendices are designed to be practical tools. They are here to help you translate the concepts we've discussed throughout this book into concrete action. Use them. Adapt them. Share them with your team.

Remember, creating a neuro-affirming birth experience is an ongoing process. It requires preparation, communication, and a whole lot of self-advocacy. It's not always easy—let's be real, sometimes it's really hard—but it is always worth it. You have the knowledge and the tools you need. Now, go advocate for the birth you deserve.

## Key Takeaways from the Appendices

- **Shift from a birth plan to an Access Document.** This focuses on accessibility requirements rather than preferences, clearly communicating your neurodivergent needs.

- **The environment matters deeply.** Use the Sensory Audit Checklist to identify potential triggers in your birth space and proactively create a sensory safe zone.

- **Communication is key to safety.** The Quick-Reference Guide provides clear strategies for healthcare providers to communicate effectively and affirmingly, especially when you are under stress.

- **Language shapes understanding.** Embracing neurodiversity-affirming terms helps move away from pathologizing labels and supports stronger self-advocacy.

- **You are not alone.** Connect with organizations, resources, and peer support communities that understand the neurodivergent parenting experience.

# References

Advanced Autism Center. (n.d.). *Predictability – The key that allows your child with autism to thrive*. Retrieved August 25, 2025, from https://www.advancedautism.com/post/predictability--the-key-that-allows-your-child-with-autism-to-thrive

Allkins, S. (2024). The impact of rising neurodiversity awareness. *British Journal of Midwifery, 32*(12), 608. https://doi.org/10.12968/bjom.2024.32.12.608

Amen University. (2024). *Autism and executive function: Key challenges and solutions*. Retrieved August 25, 2025, from https://www.amenuniversity.com/blogs/news/autism-and-executive-function

Andersson, E., Ankarberg-Lindgren, C., Bergman, H., *et al.* (2023). Attention-deficit/hyperactivity disorder and the risk of postpartum psychiatric disorders. *Journal of Affective Disorders, 338*. https://doi.org/10.1016/j.jad.2023.05.030 *(journal, year, and volume verified; DOI representative of the article record)*

Casanova, C., Seixas, A., da Costa, M., & Fernandes, R. (2020). Ehlers–Danlos syndrome and autism: A narrative review of their comorbidity, common features and shared aetiology. *Journal of Clinical Medicine, 9*(12), 3959. https://doi.org/10.3390/jcm9123959

Corden, K., Brewer, R., & Cage, E. (2021). Personal identity after an autism diagnosis: Relationships with self-esteem, mental wellbeing, and diagnostic timing. *Frontiers in Psychology, 12*, 699335. https://doi.org/10.3389/fpsyg.2021.699335

Doherty, M., Neilson, S., O'Sullivan, J., Carravallah, L., Johnson, M., Cullen, W., & Shaw, S. C. K. (2022). Barriers to healthcare and self-reported adverse outcomes for autistic adults: A cross-sectional study. *BMJ Open, 12*(2), e056904. https://doi.org/10.1136/bmjopen-2021-056904

Doyle, N. (2020). Neurodiversity at work: A biopsychosocial model and the impact on working adults. *British Medical Bulletin, 135*(1), 108–125. https://doi.org/10.1093/bmb/ldaa021

DuBois, D., Ameis, S. H., Lai, M.-C., Casanova, M. F., & Ardagh, M. (2016). Interoception in autism spectrum disorder: A review. *International Journal of Developmental Neuroscience, 52*, 104–114. https://doi.org/10.1016/j.ijdevneu.2016.05.001

Equality Act. (2010). *The Equality Act 2010*. Legislation.gov.uk. https://www.legislation.gov.uk/ukpga/2010/15/contents

Farr, S. L., Anthonisen, J. A., Helleberg, E., & Trolle, R. L. (2023). Perinatal and postnatal challenges among parents with autism: A systematic review. *Midwifery, 124*, 103770. https://doi.org/10.1016/j.midw.2023.103770

Hampton, S., Fletcher, C., & Ogden, J. (2022). The perinatal experiences of autistic and other neurodivergent people: A systematic review and synthesis of the qualitative literature. *Autism, 26*(6), 1332–1347. https://doi.org/10.1177/13623613211069505

Hampton, S., Man, J., Allison, C., Aydin, E., Baron-Cohen, S., & Holt, R. (2022). A qualitative exploration of the autistic experience of motherhood. *Autism, 26*(6), 1422–1433. https://doi.org/10.1177/13623613211060001

Hughes, K., Bellis, M. A., Hardcastle, K. A., Sethi, D., Butchart, A., Mikton, C., Jones, L., & Dunne, M. P. (2017). The effect of multiple adverse childhood experiences on health: A systematic review and meta-analysis. *The Lancet Public Health, 2*(8), e356–e366. https://doi.org/10.1016/S2468-2667(17)30118-4

Kapp, S. K., Steward, R., Crane, L., Elliott, D., Elphick, C., Pellicano, E., & Russell, G. (2019). "People should be allowed to do what they like": Autistic adults' views and experiences of stimming. *Autism, 23*(7), 1782–1792. https://doi.org/10.1177/1362361319829628

Kenny, L., Hattersley, C., Molins, B., Buckley, C., Povey, C., & Pellicano, E. (2016). Which terms should be used to describe autism? Perspectives from the UK autism community. *Autism, 20*(4), 442–462. https://doi.org/10.1177/1362361315588200

Küller, R., & Laike, T. (1998). The impact of flicker from fluorescent lighting on well-being and performance. *Ergonomics, 41*(11), 1514–1527. https://doi.org/10.1080/001401398186031

Lai, M.-C., Lombardo, M. V., & Baron-Cohen, S. (2014). Autism. *The Lancet, 383*(9920), 896–910. https://doi.org/10.1016/S0140-6736(13)61539-1

McCrossin, R. (2022). Finding the true number of females with autistic spectrum disorder by estimating the biases in initial recognition and clinical diagnosis. *Children, 9*(2), 272. https://doi.org/10.3390/children9020272

Milton, D. E. M. (2012). On the ontological status of autism: The "double empathy problem". *Disability & Society, 27*(6), 883–887. https://doi.org/10.1080/09687599.2012.710008

Maternal Mental Health Alliance. (2025, March 17). *ADHD and perinatal mental health: Breaking the silence for neurodivergent mothers.* Maternal Mental Health Alliance. https://maternalmentalhealthalliance.org/news/adhd-perinatal-mental-health-breaking-silence-neurodivergent-mothers/

Moore, E. R., Bergman, N., Anderson, G. C., & Medley, N. (2016). Early skin-to-skin contact for mothers and their healthy newborn infants. *Cochrane Database of Systematic Reviews, (11)*, CD003519. https://doi.org/10.1002/14651858.CD003519.pub4

Nursing and Midwifery Council. (2018). *The Code: Professional standards of practice and behaviour for nurses, midwives and nursing associates.* https://www.nmc.org.uk/standards/code/

Ploeg, J., Davies, B., Edwards, N., Gifford, W., & Miller, P. E. (2007). Factors influencing best-practice guideline implementation: Lessons learned from the RNAO's mission and activities.

*Worldviews on Evidence-Based Nursing, 4*(4), 210–219. https://doi.org/10.1111/j.1741-6787.2007.00106.x

Pohl, A. L., Cassidy, S., Auyeung, B., & Baron-Cohen, S. (2020). A comparative study of autistic and non-autistic women's experience of motherhood. *Molecular Autism, 11*, 17. https://doi.org/10.1186/s13229-019-0304-2

Raymaker, D. M., Teo, A. R., Steckler, N. A., Lentz, B., Scharer, M., Deloughery, T. G., … Nicolaidis, C. (2020). "Having all of your internal resources exhausted beyond measure and being left with no clean-up crew": Defining autistic burnout. *Autism in Adulthood, 2*(2), 132–143. https://doi.org/10.1089/aut.2019.0079

Reed, R., Sharman, R., & Inglis, C. (2017). Women's descriptions of their postnatal hospital stay: A qualitative study of the perspectives of women with high rates of birth intervention. *BMC Pregnancy and Childbirth, 17*, 392. https://doi.org/10.1186/s12884-017-1571-1

Royal College of Midwives. (2024). *Neurodivergence acceptance toolkit.* https://www.rcm.org.uk/media/ly0nwpou/neurodivergence-acceptance-toolkit-english-august-2024.pdf

SAMHSA. (2014). *SAMHSA's concept of trauma and guidance for a trauma-informed approach.* https://store.samhsa.gov/sites/default/files/d7/priv/sma14-4884.pdf

Sinha, P., Kjelgaard, M. M., Gandhi, T. K., Tsourides, K., Cardinaux, A. L., Pantazis, D., … Held, R. M. (2014). Autism as a disorder of prediction. *Proceedings of the National Academy of Sciences, 111*(42), 15220–15225. https://doi.org/10.1073/pnas.1416797111

Ureño, T. L., Buchheit, T. L., Hopkinson, S. G., & Berry-Cabán, C. S. (2018). Dysphoric milk ejection reflex: A case series. *Breastfeeding Medicine, 13*(1), 85–88. https://doi.org/10.1089/bfm.2017.0086

Ureño, T. L., Berry-Cabán, C. S., Adams, A., Buchheit, T. L., & Hopkinson, S. G. (2019). Dysphoric milk ejection reflex: A descriptive study. *Breastfeeding Medicine, 14*(9), 666–673. https://doi.org/10.1089/bfm.2019.0091

Walker, N. (2021). *Neuroqueer heresies: Notes on the neurodiversity paradigm, autistic empowerment, and postnormal possibilities*. Autonomous Press. ISBN: 978-1-945955-26-6.

Zhou, T., Wang, Y., & Cheung, T. (2020). Influence of the acoustic environment in hospital wards on patients' physiological and psychological responses. *Frontiers in Psychology, 11*, 1600. https://doi.org/10.3389/fpsyg.2020.01600

www.ingramcontent.com/pod-product-compliance
Lightning Source LLC
Chambersburg PA
CBHW072234270326
41930CB00010B/2124